An Introduction to Radiation Protection

Fifth edition

Alan Martin

and

Sam Harbison

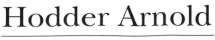
Hodder Arnold

A MEMBER OF THE HODDER HEADLINE GROUP

First published in Great Britain in 1972 by Chapman and Hall
Second edition 1979
Third edition 1986
Fourth edition 1996
This fifth edition published in 2006 by
Hodder Arnold, an imprint of Hodder Education and a member of the Hodder Headline Group,
an Hachette Livre UK Company, 338 Euston Road, London NW1 3BH

http://www.hoddereducation.com

Whilst the advice and information in this book are believed to be true and accurate at the date of going to press, neither the author[s] nor the publisher can accept any legal responsibility or liability for any errors or omissions that may be made. In particular (but without limiting the generality of the preceding disclaimer) every effort has been made to check drug dosages; however it is still possible that errors have been missed. Furthermore, dosage schedules are constantly being revised and new side-effects recognized. For these reasons the reader is strongly urged to consult the drug companies' printed instructions before administering any of the drugs recommended in this book.

British Library Cataloguing in Publication Data
A catalogue record for this book is available from the British Library

Library of Congress Cataloging-in-Publication Data
A catalog record for this book is available from the Library of Congress

ISBN: 978 0 340 885 437

2 3 4 5 6 7 8 9 10

Commissioning Editor: Philip Shaw
Production Editor: Heather Fyfe
Production Controller: Karen Tate
Cover Designer: Tim Pattinson

Typeset in 10/12 Minion by Charon Tec Ltd, Chennai, India
www.charontec.com
Printed and bound in Malta

What do you think about this book? Or any other Hodder Arnold title?
Please send your comments to www.hoddereducation.com

Dedicated to the memory of Margaret Gail Harbison

Contents

Preface

An Introduction to Radiation Protection is a comprehensive account of radiation hazards and their control. The book is intended to meet the requirements of a wide range of readers who are involved, either directly or indirectly, with ionizing radiation, including doctors, dentists, research workers, nuclear plant designers and operators. In particular, we believe that the work is suitable for the health physics monitors and technicians who are concerned with the day-to-day control of radiation hazards in nuclear power stations, research establishments, hospitals and in industry. In the UK, the generally accepted standard of training in this type of work is that set by the City and Guilds of London Institute courses in Radiation Safety Practice which are held in various centres. The chapters of the book dealing with the general aspects of health physics are aimed at this standard. Later chapters dealing with particular aspects of the subject are more detailed so that, for example, a health physics monitor in a nuclear power station or a technician in a hospital can get a deeper understanding of the problems in their own area.

When discussing legislation and regulations relating to radiation protection, we have illustrated the position by reference to the requirements in the UK. Otherwise the principles and practice set out in the book are internationally applicable. Although SI units are used throughout the book, a table of conversion factors is provided for those still using 'old' units.

Every attempt has been made to avoid detailed mathematical treatment but it has been necessary, in some areas, to use some simple mathematics. This includes squares, square roots, exponentials, logarithms and the plotting of graphs on logarithmic scales. Where a mathematical treatment is used we have tried to present it in such a way that, if the mathematics is not fully understood, it does not preclude an understanding of the chapter in general.

As far as possible each chapter is self-contained so that the reader can find all the information on a particular aspect without having to search through several chapters. The early chapters deal with basic physical principles, the nature of the hazard arising from the interaction of ionizing radiations with biological systems and the levels of radiation which are regarded as acceptable. Later chapters deal with the methods of measurement and control which are applied to attain these levels. In the second half of the book there are individual chapters on the more specialized topics of nuclear reactor health physics, problems associated with X-rays and radiography, health physics in medicine, the disposal of radioactive waste and radiological emergencies. Chapters are also presented on legislation and on the organization of health physics. Each chapter is followed by a summary in note form, in which the major points are reiterated. In addition, a number of revision questions requiring both descriptive and numerical answers are provided for the majority of chapters.

AM
SAH
London, 2006

Acknowledgements

We are pleased to acknowledge the expert help we have been given during the preparation of this edition. In particular, we are grateful to Cathy Griffiths, Consultant, and Mark Singleton of the Royal Hallamshire Hospital for their review of and helpful comments on Chapter 13. We are also indebted to Bob Anderson, Colin Partington and Rex Strong of British Nuclear Group, and John Skegg and Guy Renn of British Energy for advice and assistance in connection with protective clothing and equipment.

Although we have benefited from many helpful and constructive suggestions during the preparation of this and earlier editions, the opinions and conclusions expressed in the book are those of the authors.

The structure of matter

1

1.1 INTRODUCTION

Matter is the name given to the materials of which the Universe is composed. It exists in three physical forms: solid, liquid or gas. All matter consists of a number of simple substances called elements.

An **element** is a substance that cannot be broken down by ordinary chemical processes into simpler substances. There are 92 naturally occurring elements, examples of which are carbon, oxygen, iron and lead. Another dozen or so have been produced artificially over the past 60 years or so, the best known of which is plutonium.

In nature, elements are usually chemically linked to other elements in the form of compounds. A **compound** consists of two or more elements chemically linked in definite proportions, e.g. water, H_2O, which consists of two atoms of hydrogen and one atom of oxygen.

1.2 THE ATOM

Consider an imaginary experiment in which a quantity of some element is subjected to repeated subdivisions. Using ordinary optical instruments a stage would eventually be reached when the fragments cease to be visible. Supposing, however, that suitable tools and viewing apparatus were available, would it be possible to repeat the divisions of the original element indefinitely or would a stage be reached where the matter can no longer be subdivided?

More than 2000 years ago, the Greek philosophers considered this question. With none of our modern instruments available to them, all they could do was consider the problem in a logical manner. From this philosophical approach some of them decided that eventually a limit must be reached. They called the individual particles of matter, which could not be further subdivided, **atoms**. It was also postulated by some of the philosophers that all substances consist of these same atoms, different arrangements of the constituent atoms giving the different properties of the substances and the density being determined by how tightly the atoms are packed.

Early in the nineteenth century, an atomic theory with a scientific basis was advanced which confirmed many of the views held by the ancient philosophers. This was the atomic theory of Dalton which was able to explain the well-established but little understood chemical laws. Modern theory has diverged somewhat from Dalton's but he did establish the principle that matter consists of atoms, each element having its own characteristic atom.

1.3 THE STRUCTURE OF THE ATOM

It is now known that atoms are not solid, indivisible objects as the Greek philosophers believed but are composed of even smaller particles. These particles, from which all atoms are constructed, are called **protons**, **neutrons** and **electrons**.

The **proton** (p) carries a positive electrical charge of magnitude one unit on the nuclear scale, and a mass of approximately one atomic mass unit (u).

The **electron** (e^-) has a negative electrical charge of the same magnitude as the proton's positive charge. It has a mass of 1/1840 u, which, for most purposes, is neglected in considering the mass of the atom.

The **neutron** (n) is often regarded as a close combination of a proton and an electron. It is electrically neutral and has a mass of approximately one atomic mass unit. In the text and in illustrations the neutron is generally treated as a fundamental particle, in common with normal usage.

The neutrons and protons of an atom form a central core or nucleus, around which the electrons rotate in various orbits, normally referred to as shells. The shell closest to the nucleus can contain a maximum of two electrons, while the second can have up to eight, with progressively greater numbers in the outer shells. The inner shell is known as the **K shell**, the second is called the **L shell**, the third the **M shell**, and so on. The maximum numbers of electrons in the K, L, M and N shells are 2, 8, 18 and 32 respectively. For example, the atomic system of zinc, illustrated in Fig. 1.1, has 30 electrons arranged in four shells.

Each atom normally has the same number of protons as electrons. This means that the total positive charge on the nucleus is equal to the total negative charge of the atomic

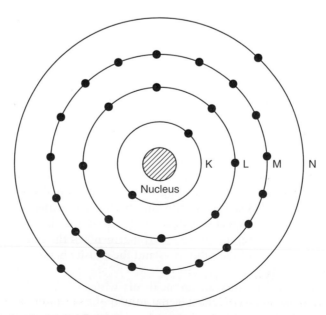

FIGURE 1.1 The atomic system of zinc.

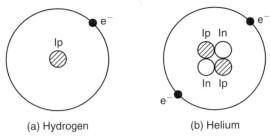

(a) Hydrogen   (b) Helium

FIGURE 1.2 The atomic systems of hydrogen and helium.

electrons, and so the atom is normally electrically neutral. Two simple atoms, those of hydrogen and helium, are illustrated in Fig. 1.2. Note that this particular hydrogen atom is the only atom that does not contain neutrons.

1.4 ELEMENTS AND ATOMIC NUMBER

The number of protons in an atom is called the atomic number and is represented by the symbol Z:

Atomic number (Z) = number of protons

For example

hydrogen has 1 proton, $Z = 1$
helium has 2 protons, $Z = 2$

It is the number of protons in an atom that determines its chemical properties and so defines the element.

Thus:

all atoms with an atomic number of 1 are hydrogen atoms (chemical symbol H)
all atoms with an atomic number of 2 are helium atoms (He)
all atoms with an atomic number of 3 are lithium atoms (Li)
all atoms with an atomic number of 4 are beryllium atoms (Be)
all atoms with an atomic number of 5 are boron atoms (B)
all atoms with an atomic number of 6 are carbon atoms (C) …, etc.,

up to the heaviest naturally-occurring element, uranium (U), which has an atomic number of 92. About a dozen or so elements of higher atomic number have been artificially produced in the past half century or so. They are all unstable and can only be made under special conditions which are not found naturally on Earth.

1.5 ISOTOPES AND MASS NUMBER

Although all the atoms of a particular element contain the same number of protons, they may occur with different numbers of neutrons. This means that an element can have

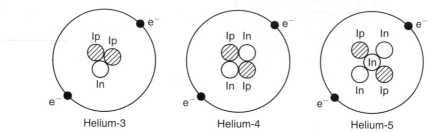

FIGURE 1.3 The three isotopes of helium.

several types of atom. For example, hydrogen can occur with 0, 1 or 2 neutrons in its nucleus and the three different types of atom are called **isotopes** of hydrogen.

The mass of an atom is fixed by the number of protons and neutrons, if the very small mass of the atomic electrons is neglected. The sum of the number of protons plus the number of neutrons is called the **mass number** and is represented by the symbol A:

$$\text{Mass number } (A) = \text{number of protons} + \text{number of neutrons}$$

For example, the helium atom in Fig. 1.2b contains 2 protons and 2 neutrons and so has a mass number of 4. Helium can also occur with 1 or 3 neutrons in the nucleus, as shown in Fig. 1.3. These three isotopes are normally referred to as helium-3, helium-4 and helium-5, which are often shortened to He-3, He-4 and He-5.

In symbolic form, an isotope can also be written as $_Z^A$X, where X is the symbol for the element and A and Z are the atomic number and mass number, respectively. In this format, helium-3 is written $_2^3$He. Strictly, showing the atomic number is unnecessary because the name of the element defines the atomic number and in most cases it is sufficient to write this as ^{3}He. Throughout this text, in using this notation the atomic number is included where it assists an understanding of the topic.

Considering another example, the element phosphorus (P) has an atomic number of 15 (i.e. each atom contains 15 protons), but it can occur with different numbers of neutrons. In other words, there are several isotopes of phosphorus, as shown below.

$_{15}^{28}$P has 15 protons and 13 neutrons ($Z = 15, A = 28$)

$_{15}^{29}$P has 15 protons and 14 neutrons ($Z = 15, A = 29$)

$_{15}^{30}$P has 15 protons and 15 neutrons ($Z = 15, A = 30$)

$_{15}^{31}$P has 15 protons and 16 neutrons ($Z = 15, A = 31$)

$_{15}^{32}$P has 15 protons and 17 neutrons ($Z = 15, A = 32$)

$_{15}^{33}$P has 15 protons and 18 neutrons ($Z = 15, A = 33$)

$_{15}^{34}$P has 15 protons and 19 neutrons ($Z = 15, A = 34$)

It is important to note that all the isotopes of a given element are **chemically** identical, since the chemical properties are determined by the atomic number of the element.

Most elements occur naturally as a mixture of isotopes, and other isotopes may be produced by bombarding a naturally occurring isotope with nuclear particles, for example by neutrons in a nuclear reactor. These artificially produced isotopes are unstable and will eventually disintegrate with the emission of a secondary particle (see Chapter 2).

Apart from the few lightest elements the number of neutrons exceeds the number of protons in an atom. The difference becomes greater as Z increases, as illustrated by the following examples:

$$^{4}_{2}\text{He has 2 protons and 2 neutrons}$$

$$^{31}_{15}\text{P has 15 protons and 16 neutrons}$$

$$^{65}_{30}\text{Zn has 30 protons and 35 neutrons}$$

$$^{238}_{92}\text{U has 92 protons and 146 neutrons}$$

Data on the known isotopes of all the elements, both naturally occurring and artificially produced, have been arranged systematically in a table known as the **chart of the nuclides** which will be discussed in more detail in Chapter 2. The term **nuclide** means any isotope of any element.

1.6 ANCIENT AND MODERN THEORIES

It will now be seen that the ancient Greek philosophers were remarkably close to the truth in their theory that all substances are constituted from the same basic particles. However, instead of being different arrangements of only one type of particle, different substances appear to result from various combinations of protons, neutrons and electrons. It is now known that protons and neutrons are made up of still smaller particles called quarks and there is some evidence of apparently more fundamental particles, so that the ancient Greeks may yet prove to have been right in their conjecture that there is one fundamental particle that is the basis for all others.

SUMMARY OF CHAPTER

Element: material whose atoms all have the same number of protons.
u: atomic mass unit.
Proton: atomic particle, mass 1 u, charge $+1$ unit.
Electron: atomic particle, mass 1/1840 u, charge -1 unit.
Neutron: close combination of proton and electron, mass 1 u, electrically neutral.
Atom: central nucleus of protons and neutrons, around which electrons rotate in orbits.
Atomic number (Z): number of protons.
Mass number (A): number of protons plus number of neutrons.
Isotope: one of several nuclides with the same atomic number.
Notation: there are several ways of referring to an isotope: for example, phosphorus-32, P-32, $^{32}_{15}\text{P}$ and ^{32}P.
Nuclide: a nuclear species.

REVISION QUESTIONS

1. Following the illustration in Fig. 1.1, draw an atom of each of the following nuclides:

$$^{4}_{2}\text{He}, \quad ^{6}_{3}\text{Li}, \quad ^{7}_{3}\text{Li}, \quad ^{8}_{4}\text{Be}$$

2. The nuclide cobalt-60 may be written $^{60}_{27}$Co. How many protons, electrons and neutrons are there in this type of atom?

3. What are the masses and charges on the atomic scale of protons, electrons and neutrons?

4. Which atomic property determines the chemical behaviour of an element?

5. Explain what is meant by the term isotope. Give some examples.

Radioactivity and radiation

2.1 INTRODUCTION

It is found that a few naturally occurring substances consist of atoms which are unstable – that is, they undergo spontaneous transformation into more stable product atoms. Such substances are said to be **radioactive** and the transformation process is known as **radioactive decay**. Radioactive decay is usually accompanied by the emission of radiation in the form of charged particles and gamma (γ)-rays.

The fact that some elements are naturally radioactive was first realized by Becquerel in 1896. He observed blackening of photographic emulsions in the vicinity of a uranium compound. This was subsequently attributed to the effect of radiation being emitted by the uranium. In the following 10 years the experimental work of Rutherford and Soddy, Pierre and Marie Curie and others established the fact that some types of nuclei are not completely stable. These unstable nuclei decay and emit radiations of three main types, called **alpha**, **beta** and **gamma** radiation.

2.2 ALPHA, BETA AND GAMMA RADIATION

Alpha (α) radiation was shown by Rutherford and Royds to consist of helium nuclei which themselves consist of two protons and two neutrons. These four particles are bound together so tightly that the α particle behaves in many situations as if it were a fundamental particle. An α particle has a mass of 4 u and carries two units of positive charge.

Beta (β) radiation consists of high-speed electrons which originate in the nucleus. These 'nuclear electrons' have identical properties to the atomic electrons, that is they have a mass of 1/1840 u and carry one unit of negative charge. Another type of β radiation was discovered by C. D. Anderson in 1932. This consists of particles of the same mass as the electron but having one unit of positive charge; it is known as positron radiation. Although less important from a radiation protection viewpoint than negative β particles, a knowledge of positrons is necessary to understand certain radioactive decay mechanisms. Beta radiation is signified β^- (electrons) or β^+ (positrons). In everyday use the term β radiation normally refers to the negative type, β^-.

Gamma (γ) radiation belongs to a class known as electromagnetic radiation. This type of radiation is often described as consisting of photons which are in some ways analogous to α or β particles. However, the photons do not have mass but consist of quanta or packets of energy transmitted in the form of a wave motion. Other well-known members of this class of radiation are radio waves and visible light. The amount of energy in each quantum is related to the wavelength of the radiation. The energy is inversely proportional to the wavelength, which means that the shorter the wavelength the higher the energy. Mathematically, this is written as $E \propto 1/\lambda$, where E is the energy of the quantum or photon of electromagnetic radiation and λ is its wavelength. Another class of electromagnetic radiation which is in most respects identical to γ radiation is known as X radiation. The essential difference between the two types of radiation lies in their origin. Whereas γ-rays result from changes in the nucleus, X-rays are emitted when atomic electrons undergo a change in orbit.

The wavelength of electromagnetic radiation varies over a very wide range, as illustrated in Table 2.1.

Table 2.1 Wavelengths of electromagnetic radiations

Type of radiation	Wavelength, λ (m)
Radio waves, long wave	1500
Radio waves, VHF	3
Visible light	10^{-6} to 10^{-7}
X-rays, 50 keV energy	2.5×10^{-11}
Gamma-rays, 1 MeV energy	1.2×10^{-12}

All electromagnetic radiations travel through free space with the same velocity of 3×10^8 m/s. Their velocity decreases in dense media but in air the decrease is negligible.

2.3 THE ELECTRONVOLT

Radiation energy is expressed in **electronvolts** (eV). One electronvolt is the energy gained by an electron in passing through an electrical potential of 1 volt.

For example, in the cathode ray tube of a television receiver, electrons are accelerated from the electron gun to the screen through an electrical potential of about 10 000 volts. The electrons therefore have an energy of 10 000 eV when they strike the screen.

The electronvolt is a very small unit so radiation energies are usually expressed in **kilo** (1000) or **mega** (1 000 000) electronvolts:

One kiloelectronvolt = 1 keV = 1000 eV
One megaelectronvolt = 1 MeV = 1000 keV = 1 000 000 eV

Even if the radiation being considered is not β (electron) radiation, it is still possible to express its energy in terms of the electronvolt.

The energy of a particle depends on its mass and velocity, e.g., the kinetic energy (E_K) of a particle of mass m travelling with velocity v, much smaller than the velocity of light, is given by the equation

$$E_K = \tfrac{1}{2}mv^2$$

(A correction is necessary for particles having velocities approaching the velocity of light.) A small particle such as an electron requires a much higher velocity than, say, an α particle to have the same kinetic energy.

In the case of electromagnetic radiation, the energy is inversely proportional to the wavelength of the radiation. Thus radiations with short wavelengths have higher energies than radiations with longer wavelengths.

2.4 THE MECHANISM OF RADIOACTIVE DECAY

The nuclei of the heavier elements found in nature are so large that they are slightly unstable. For example, the isotope uranium-238 has 92 protons and 146 neutrons. To achieve greater stability the nucleus may emit an α particle, so reducing its numbers of protons and neutrons to 90 and 144, respectively. This means that the nucleus now has an atomic number (Z) of 90 instead of 92 and so is no longer a uranium nucleus. It is now an isotope of the element thorium (Th) with atomic number 90 and mass number 234, namely thorium-234. This decay process may be represented as follows:

$$\ce{^{238}_{92}U} \longrightarrow \ce{^{4}_{2}\alpha} + \ce{^{234}_{90}Th}$$

or, more commonly,

$$\ce{^{238}_{92}U} \xrightarrow{\alpha} \ce{^{234}_{90}Th}$$

Another example of this process is the decay of polonium-218 (^{218}Po) by α emission to lead-214 (^{214}Pb):

$$\ce{^{218}_{84}Po} \xrightarrow{\alpha} \ce{^{214}_{82}Pb}$$

It was pointed out in Chapter 1 that there are more neutrons than protons in heavy nuclei. Alpha emission reduces the number of each by two but the proportionate reduction is considerably less for neutrons than for protons. In the ^{238}U decay process, the number of protons is reduced by two out of 92 whereas the number of neutrons is reduced by two out of 146, which is significantly less. The effect of α emission is therefore to produce neutron-rich nuclei which are still unstable. The nucleus does not simply eject a neutron (or neutrons) to correct this instability. Instead, one of the neutrons in the nucleus changes into a proton by emitting a β particle, i.e. a high-speed electron:

$$\ce{^{1}_{0}n} \longrightarrow \ce{^{1}_{1}p} + \beta^{-}$$

This phenomenon is known as **β emission**. In the case of ^{234}Th, formed by the α-decay of ^{238}U, the nucleus further decays by β emission to protactinium-234 (^{234}Pa):

$$\ce{^{234}_{90}Th} \longrightarrow \ce{^{234}_{91}Pa} + \beta^{-}$$

or

$$\ce{^{234}_{90}Th} \xrightarrow{\beta^{-}} \ce{^{234}_{91}Pa}$$

Considering again polonium-218, the complete decay is:

$$\underset{84}{^{218}}\text{Po} \xrightarrow{\alpha} \underset{82}{^{214}}\text{Pb} \xrightarrow{\beta^-} \underset{83}{^{214}}\text{Bi}$$

The resulting atom is bismuth-214, which is also unstable and so further α- and β-decay processes occur until a stable atom is produced.

Electrons emitted during β-decay have a continuous distribution in energy, ranging from zero to a maximum energy E_{max} which is characteristic of the particular nucleus. The most probable β energy is about $1/3E_{max}$ (see Fig. 2.1).

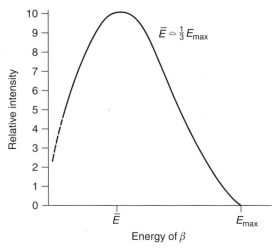

FIGURE 2.1 Typical β spectrum.

In most cases, after the emission of an α or β particle, the nucleus rearranges itself slightly, releasing energy by γ **emission.**

Two other decay processes should also be mentioned, namely **positron emission** and **electron capture.** In positron emission, a proton in the nucleus ejects a positive electron (β^+) and so becomes a neutron:

$$\underset{1}{^{1}}\text{p} \longrightarrow \underset{0}{^{1}}\text{n} + \beta^+$$

For example, sodium-22 (Na-22) decays by positron emission to Neon-22:

$$\underset{11}{^{22}}\text{Na} \xrightarrow{\beta^+} \underset{10}{^{22}}\text{Ne}$$

Electron capture is a process in which an electron from an inner orbit is captured by the nucleus resulting in the conversion of a proton to a neutron:

$$\underset{1}{^{1}}\text{p} + e^- \longrightarrow \underset{0}{^{1}}\text{n}$$

A rearrangement of atomic electrons then causes the emission of X-rays.

2.5 NATURAL RADIOACTIVE SERIES

Apart from ^{22}Na, the above examples of radioactive decay are all naturally occurring radioactive substances and belong to the so-called **natural radioactive series**. There are three natural radioactive series, called the thorium, uranium–radium and actinium series (see Table 2.2). Also included in this table is the neptunium series which does not occur in nature because the half-life ($T_{1/2}$, see Section 2.7) of its longest-lived member is only 2.2×10^6 years, which is much less than the age of the Earth (about 3×10^9 years).

Table 2.2 Natural radioactive series

Series name	Final stable nucleus	Longest-lived member
Thorium	^{208}Pb	^{232}Th ($T_{1/2} = 1.39 \times 10^{10}$ years)
Uranium–radium	^{206}Pb	^{238}U ($T_{1/2} = 4.50 \times 10^9$ years)
Actinium	^{207}Pb	^{235}U ($T_{1/2} = 8.52 \times 10^8$ years)
Neptunium	^{209}Bi	^{237}Np ($T_{1/2} = 2.20 \times 10^6$ years)

The term series is used because an atom undergoes a succession of radioactive transformations until it reaches a stable state. In the thorium series, the atom is initially thorium-232 and undergoes a series of radioactive decays as follows:

$$^{232}_{90}\text{Th} \xrightarrow{\alpha} {}^{228}_{88}\text{Ra} \xrightarrow{\beta^-} {}^{228}_{89}\text{Ac} \xrightarrow{\beta^-} {}^{228}_{90}\text{Th} \xrightarrow{\alpha} {}^{224}_{88}\text{Ra} \xrightarrow{\alpha}$$

$$^{220}_{86}\text{Rn} \xrightarrow{\alpha} {}^{216}_{84}\text{Po} \xrightarrow{\alpha} {}^{212}_{82}\text{Pb} \xrightarrow{\beta^-} {}^{212}_{83}\text{Bi} \xrightarrow{\beta^-} {}^{212}_{84}\text{Po} \xrightarrow{\alpha} {}^{208}_{82}\text{Pb}$$

The half-lives of these members of the decay series range from 0.15 s for polonium-216 to about 1.4×10^{10} years for thorium-232.

2.6 INDUCED RADIOACTIVITY

Lighter elements may be made radioactive by bombarding them with nuclear particles. One such process involves the bombardment of stable nuclei of an element by neutrons in a nuclear reactor. A neutron may be captured by a nucleus, with the emission of a γ photon. This is known as a neutron, gamma (n, γ) reaction. The resulting atom is usually unstable because of the excess neutron and will eventually decay by β-emission.

Thus if the stable isotope cobalt-59 is bombarded or irradiated with neutrons, atoms of the radioactive isotope cobalt-60 are produced. These atoms will eventually undergo β-decay and become atoms of the stable isotope nickel-60. This process is written as:

$$^{59}_{27}\text{Co}(n, \gamma)^{60}_{27}\text{Co} \xrightarrow{\beta^-} {}^{60}_{28}\text{Ni}$$

There are various other activation and decay processes which will be discussed later.

2.7 THE UNIT OF RADIOACTIVITY

The decay of a radioactive sample is statistical in nature and it is impossible to predict when any particular atom will disintegrate. The consequence of this random behaviour of radioactive atoms is that the radioactive decay law is exponential in nature, and is expressed mathematically as:

$$N_t = N_0 e^{-\lambda t}$$

where N_0 is the number of nuclei present initially, N_t is the number of nuclei present at time t and λ is the radioactive decay constant.

The **half-life** ($T_{1/2}$) of a radioactive species is the time required for one-half of the nuclei in a sample to decay. It is obtained by putting $N_t = N_0/2$ in the above equation:

$$N_0/2 = N_0 e^{-\lambda T_{1/2}}$$

Dividing across by N_0 and taking logs

$$\log_e(\tfrac{1}{2}) = -\lambda T_{1/2}$$

Now

$$\log_e(\tfrac{1}{2}) = -\log_e(2)$$

and so

$$T_{1/2} = \frac{\log_e 2}{\lambda} = \frac{0.693}{\lambda}$$

Since the disintegration rate, or **activity**, of the sample is proportional to the number of unstable nuclei, this also varies exponentially with time in accordance with the equation

$$A_t = A_0 e^{-\lambda t}$$

This relationship is illustrated in Fig. 2.2 which shows the variation of sample activity with time. In one half-life the activity decays to $\tfrac{1}{2}A_0$, in two half-lives to $\tfrac{1}{4}A_0$, and so on. The half-life of a particular radioactive isotope is constant and its measurement assists in the identification of radioactive samples of unknown composition. This method can only be applied to isotopes whose disintegration rates change appreciably over reasonable counting periods. At the other end of the scale, the isotope must have a long enough half-life to allow some measurements to be made before it all disintegrates. To determine extremely short and extremely long half-lives, more elaborate means must be used. Half-lives range from about 10^{-14} years (^{212}Po) to about 10^{17} years (^{209}Bi), which represents a factor of 10^{31}.

For many years, the unit of radioactivity was the **curie** (Ci), but this has now been generally replaced by the SI unit, the **becquerel** (Bq). The curie was originally related to the activity of 1 g of radium but the definition was later standardized as 3.7×10^{10} nuclear disintegrations (dis) per second, which is almost the same:

$$1 \text{ curie (Ci)} = 3.7 \times 10^{10} \text{ dis/s or } 2.22 \times 10^{12} \text{ dis/min}$$

The becquerel is defined as one nuclear disintegration per second and, compared with the curie, it is a very small unit. In practice, most radioactive sources are much larger than

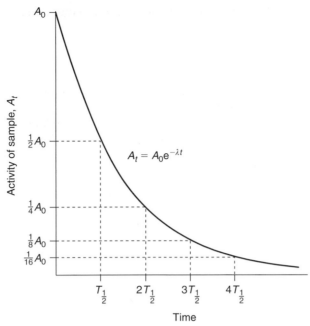

FIGURE 2.2 Variation of activity with time.

the becquerel and the following multiplying prefixes are used to describe them:

$$
\begin{aligned}
\text{1 becquerel (Bq)} &= \text{1 dis/s} \\
\text{1 kilobecquerel (kBq)} &= 10^3 \text{ Bq} = 10^3 \text{ dis/s} \\
\text{1 megabecquerel (MBq)} &= 10^6 \text{ Bq} = 10^6 \text{ dis/s} \\
\text{1 gigabecquerel (GBq)} &= 10^9 \text{ Bq} = 10^9 \text{ dis/s} \\
\text{1 terabecquerel (TBq)} &= 10^{12} \text{ Bq} = 10^{12} \text{ dis/s} \\
\text{1 petabecquerel (PBq)} &= 10^{15} \text{ Bq} = 10^{15} \text{ dis/s}
\end{aligned}
$$

For simplicity, in this text only Bq, MBq and TBq have been used.

As explained earlier, a disintegration usually involves the emission of a charged particle (α or β). This may be accompanied, although not always, by one or more γ-emissions. Some nuclides emit only X or γ radiation.

2.8 THE NUCLIDE CHART

The **nuclide chart** is a compilation of information on all known stable and unstable nuclides and a portion of it is reproduced in Fig. 2.3.

In the chart, each horizontal line represents an element and the squares on that line represent the nuclides or isotopes of the element. Relevant information regarding the nuclide is printed inside the square. Stable, naturally radioactive and artificial nuclides are differentiated by the use of different colours or shading of the squares. In each case the symbol and mass number are shown as well as the natural abundance of the isotope. For radioactive isotopes the half-life, the mode or modes of decay, and the main energies of

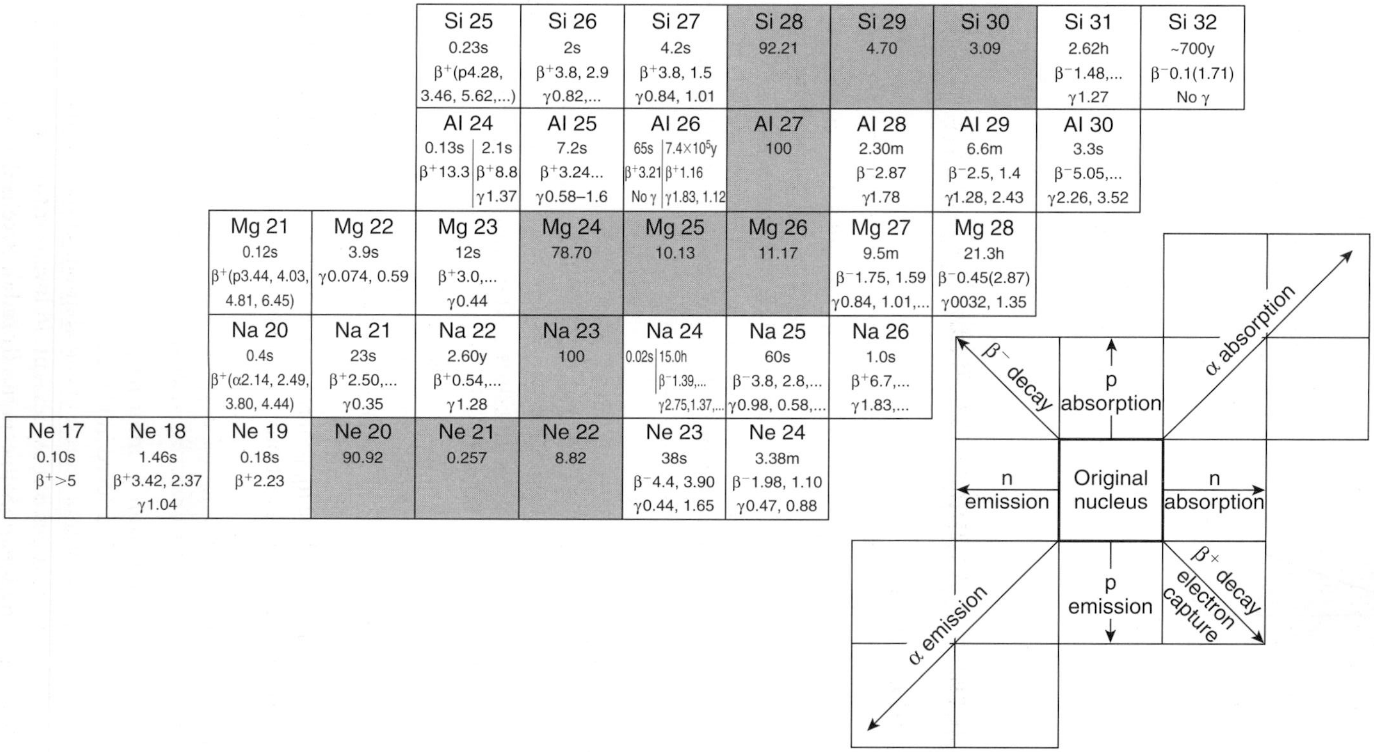

Nuclide chart entries:

Si
- Si 25 — 0.23s — β^+(p4.28, 3.46, 5.62....)
- Si 26 — 2s — β^+3.8, 2.9 γ0.82....
- Si 27 — 4.2s — β^+3.8, 1.5 γ0.84, 1.01
- Si 28 — 92.21
- Si 29 — 4.70
- Si 30 — 3.09
- Si 31 — 2.62h — β^-1.48,.... γ1.27
- Si 32 — ~700y — β^-0.1(1.71) No γ

Al
- Al 24 — 0.13s | 2.1s — β^+13.3 | β^+8.8 γ1.37
- Al 25 — 7.2s — β^+3.24... γ0.58–1.6
- Al 26 — 65s | 7.4×10^{5}y — β^+3.21 | β^+1.16 — No γ | γ1.83, 1.12
- Al 27 — 100
- Al 28 — 2.30m — β^-2.87 γ1.78
- Al 29 — 6.6m — β^-2.5, 1.4 γ1.28, 2.43
- Al 30 — 3.3s — β^-5.05,.... γ2.26, 3.52

Mg
- Mg 21 — 0.12s — β^+(p3.44, 4.03, 4.81, 6.45)
- Mg 22 — 3.9s — γ0.074, 0.59
- Mg 23 — 12s — β^+3.0.... γ0.44
- Mg 24 — 78.70
- Mg 25 — 10.13
- Mg 26 — 11.17
- Mg 27 — 9.5m — β^-1.75, 1.59 γ0.84, 1.01,....
- Mg 28 — 21.3h — β^-0.45(2.87) γ0032, 1.35

Na
- Na 20 — 0.4s — β^+(α2.14, 2.49, 3.80, 4.44)
- Na 21 — 23s — β^+2.50.... γ0.35
- Na 22 — 2.60y — β^+0.54.... γ1.28
- Na 23 — 100
- Na 24 — 15.0h | 0.02s — β^-1.39... γ2.75,1.37...
- Na 25 — 60s — β^-3.8, 2.8.... γ0.98, 0.58....
- Na 26 — 1.0s — β^+6.7,.... γ1.83,....

Ne
- Ne 17 — 0.10s — β^+>5
- Ne 18 — 1.46s — β^+3.42, 2.37 γ1.04
- Ne 19 — 0.18s — β^+2.23
- Ne 20 — 90.92
- Ne 21 — 0.257
- Ne 22 — 8.82
- Ne 23 — 38s — β^-4.4, 3.90 γ0.44, 1.65
- Ne 24 — 3.38m — β^-1.98, 1.10 γ0.47, 0.88

Legend:
- Original nucleus
- n absorption
- p absorption
- p emission
- n emission
- β^- decay
- β^+ decay electron capture
- α absorption
- α emission

FIGURE 2.3 A portion of the nuclide chart.

the emitted particles or γ-rays are shown. In the chart illustrated in Fig. 2.3, all the nuclides on the same horizontal line have the same atomic number, while all nuclides with the same mass number lie on a 45° diagonal line, running from upper left to lower right. Many nuclide charts contain additional information which has been omitted from the sample chart shown in Fig. 2.3 for the sake of clarity.

The nuclide chart can be used to obtain rapid information on the products of various nuclear reactions. For example, a (n, γ) reaction on sodium-23 (^{23}Na) produces sodium-24 (^{24}Na). This ^{24}Na decays with a half-life of 15.0 h by emitting β^- particles of maximum energy 1.39 MeV and γ-rays of 2.75 MeV and 1.37 MeV. The nucleus resulting from the decay of ^{24}Na is magnesium-24 (^{24}Mg) which is stable.

It is obvious that, even in the simplified form shown in Fig. 2.3, the nuclide chart is an extremely valuable source of information on the properties of both stable and unstable nuclides.

2.9 INTERACTION OF RADIATION WITH MATTER

2.9.1 Charged particles

Both α and β particles lose energy mainly through interactions with atomic electrons in the absorbing medium. The energy transferred to the electrons causes them either to be excited to a higher energy level (excitation) or separated entirely from the parent atom (ionization). Another important effect is that when charged particles are slowed down very rapidly they emit energy in the form of X-rays. This is known as **bremsstrahlung** (braking radiation) and is only of practical importance in the case of β radiation.

2.9.2 X and γ radiations

X and γ radiations interact with matter through a variety of alternative mechanisms, the three most important of which are the **photoelectric effect**, **Compton scattering** and **pair-production**. In the photoelectric effect all the energy of an X- or γ-photon is transferred to an atomic electron which is ejected from its parent atom. The photon is, in this case, completely absorbed. Conversely, when Compton scattering occurs, only part of the energy of the photon is transferred to an atomic electron. The scattered photon then continues with reduced energy.

In the intense electric field close to a charged particle, usually a nucleus, an energetic γ-photon may be converted into a positron–electron pair. This is pair-production and the two resulting particles share the available energy.

Thus, all three interactions result in the photon energy being transferred to atomic electrons which subsequently lose energy as described in Section 2.9.1.

2.9.3 Neutrons

Neutrons are uncharged and cannot cause ionization directly. As with γ radiation, neutrons ultimately transfer their energy to charged particles. In addition, a neutron may be captured by a nucleus, usually resulting in γ-emission. These processes are described in greater detail in Chapter 8.

Table 2.3 summarizes the types of interactions of nuclear radiations with matter.

Table 2.3   Interactions of nuclear radiations

Radiation	Process	Remarks
Alpha	Collisions with atomic electrons	Leads to excitation and ionization
Beta	(a) Collisions with atomic electrons	Leads to excitation and ionization
	(b) Slowing-down in field of nucleus	Leads to emission of bremsstrahlung
X and γ radiation	(a) Photoelectric effect	Photon is completely absorbed
	(b) Compton effect	Only part of the photon energy
	(c) Pair-production	is absorbed
Neutron	(a) Elastic scattering	
	(b) Inelastic scattering	Discussed in Chapter 8
	(c) Capture processes	

2.10 PENETRATING POWERS OF NUCLEAR RADIATIONS

The α particle is a massive particle (by nuclear standards) and travels relatively slowly through matter. It thus has a high probability of interacting with atoms along its path and will give up some of its energy during each of these interactions. As a consequence, α particles lose their energy very rapidly and only travel very short distances in dense media.

Beta particles are very much smaller than α particles and travel much faster. Therefore, they undergo fewer interactions per unit length of track and so give up their energy more slowly than α particles. This means that β particles travel further in dense media than α particles.

Gamma radiation loses its energy mainly by interacting with atomic electrons. It travels very large distances even in dense media and is very difficult to absorb completely.

Neutrons give up their energy through a variety of interactions, the relative importances of which are dependent on the neutron energy. For this reason it is common practice to divide neutrons into at least three energy groups: fast, intermediate and thermal. Neutrons are very penetrating and will travel large distances even in dense media.

In Table 2.4 the properties and ranges of the various nuclear radiations are summarized. The ranges are only approximate since they depend on the energy of the radiation.

Table 2.4   Properties of nuclear radiations

Radiation	Mass (u)	Charge	Range in air	Range in tissue
Alpha	4	+2	0.03 m	0.04 mm
Beta	1/1840	−1 (positron +1)	3 m	5 mm
X, γ radiation	0	0	Very large	Through body
Fast neutron	1	0	Very large	Through body
Thermal neutron	1	0	Very large	0.15 m

SUMMARY OF CHAPTER

Radioactive decay: transformation of an unstable substance into a more stable form, usually accompanied by the emission of charged particles and γ-rays.

Alpha (α) radiation: helium nuclei, 2p + 2n, mass 4 u, charge +2 units.

Beta (β) radiation: high-speed electrons which originate in the nucleus, mass $1/1840$ u, charge -1 (electron) or $+1$ (positron).
Gamma (γ) radiation: electromagnetic radiation, very short wavelength, $E \propto 1/\lambda$, mass 0, charge 0.
Electronvolt: energy gained by an electron in passing through an electric potential of 1 V.

$$10^6 \text{ eV} \equiv 10^3 \text{ keV} \equiv 1 \text{ MeV}$$

Natural radioactive series: consist of naturally occurring radioactive substances; the three series are thorium, uranium–radium and actinium.
Induced radioactivity: radioactivity caused by bombarding stable atoms with nuclear particles, for example by neutrons in a nuclear reactor.
Radioactive decay law: $N_t = N_0 e^{-\lambda t}$.
Half-life: time required for one half of the nuclei of a radioactive species to decay:

$$T_{\frac{1}{2}} = \frac{0.693}{\lambda}$$

Curie (Ci): former unit of radioactivity defined as 3.7×10^{10} dis/s

$$1 \text{ Ci} \equiv 10^3 \text{ mCi} \equiv 10^6 \text{ } \mu\text{Ci}$$

Becquerel (Bq): SI unit of radioactivity, defined as 1 dis/s

$$1 \text{ TBq} \equiv 10^6 \text{ MBq} \equiv 10^{12} \text{ Bq}$$

Nuclide chart: compilation of data on all known nuclides.
Alpha particles lose energy in matter through excitation and ionization.
Beta particles lose energy by:

1. excitation and ionization of atomic electrons,
2. rapid slowing down with emission of bremsstrahlung.

Gamma-photons lose energy through:

1. photoelectric effect,
2. Compton effect,
3. pair-production.

Neutrons lose energy through:

1. elastic scatter,
2. inelastic scatter,
3. capture reactions.

REVISION QUESTIONS

1. Explain the difference between radioactivity and radiation.
2. Name the products of the following radioactive decay processes:
    (a) α-decay of uranium-238, $^{238}_{92}\text{U}$,
    (b) β^--decay of tritium, ^3_1H,
    (c) β^+-decay of copper-62, $^{62}_{29}\text{Cu}$.

3. Explain why there are only three naturally occurring radioactive series.
4. Estimate the half-life of a radioactive sample by plotting a graph of the following series of measurements:

Time (min)	0	1	2	3	4	5	6	7	8
Activity (counts/min)	–	820	605	447	330	243	180	133	98

5. Express the following activities in megabecquerels (MBq):
   (a) 5×10^6 dis/s,
   (b) 750 kBq,
   (c) 1.3 GBq,
   (d) 6×10^7 dis/min.
6. Why is an α-decay usually followed by a β^--decay?
7. Using a nuclide chart, write down the product or sequence of products which would result from a (n, γ) capture in the following nuclei:

$$^{59}_{27}\text{Fe}, \quad ^{23}_{11}\text{Na}, \quad ^{239}_{94}\text{Pu}$$

Radiation units

3.1 ABSORPTION OF ENERGY

Just as heat and light transfer energy from the Sun to the Earth and the atmosphere, so nuclear radiation transfers energy from a source to an absorbing medium. The source of nuclear radiation may be radioactive atoms or equipment such as X-ray machines. The effect of absorbing the more familiar types of radiation, such as heat, is to raise the temperature of the absorbing medium. If this medium is the human body, or part of it, the rise in temperature is sensed and, if it becomes excessive, avoiding action can be taken by sheltering under a sunshade (shielding), for example, or by moving further away from a fire (distance). However, a dose of γ radiation or other nuclear radiation large enough to be lethal to a human being would increase the body temperature by less than one-thousandth of one degree centigrade. The body is therefore unable to sense even very high intensities of these types of radiation.

Nuclear radiation differs from heat and other types of radiation in that each individual particle or photon has a sufficiently high energy to cause ionization. The high energy is due to the very high velocity of the particles or the short wavelength of the X and γ radiation.

3.2 IONIZATION

Ionization is the removal of an orbital electron from an atom. Since the electron has a negative charge, the atom is consequently left positively charged. The atom and the electron, so separated, are known as an **ion pair**, that is, a positive ion (the atom minus one electron) and a negative ion (the electron). The absorption of radiation in a medium results, then, in the production of ion pairs in the medium. A small amount of energy is required to cause ionization, so that in producing ion pairs, the particles or photons of radiation lose energy to the medium. Figure 3.1 shows the ionization of a helium atom by an α particle.

Normally, positive and negative ions recombine to form neutral atoms and the energy originally given to the ion pair is converted into heat energy. If the absorbing medium is a gas, such as air, the ions can be prevented from recombining by applying an electric field. This is done by applying a voltage between two plates (electrodes) with a gas gap between them. Figure 3.2 shows such a system, known as an ionization chamber, in which ion pairs are being produced along the track of an α particle. If the applied voltage is sufficiently high, negative ions produced in the volume between the electrodes are attracted to the

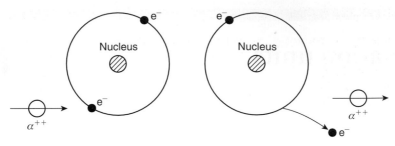

FIGURE 3.1 Ionization of a helium atom by an α particle.

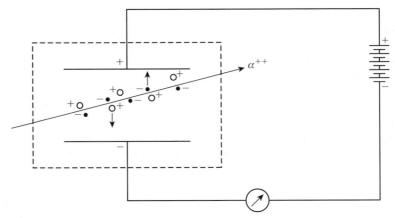

FIGURE 3.2 Ionization chamber system.

positive electrode and positive ions to the negative electrode. The flow of ions to the respective electrodes constitutes an electrical current and since this is proportional to the intensity of radiation, ion chambers provide a means of measuring radiation. It should be realized that, although only a few ion pairs are shown in the figure, in the case of β particles, several hundreds of ion pairs are formed per centimetre of track in air and, in the case of α particles, some tens of thousands.

In a medium such as water (of which the human body is largely composed) ionization can lead to breakdown of water molecules and the formation of chemical forms that are damaging to biological material. The harmful effects of radiation on the human system, which are described in Chapter 4, are largely attributable to such chemical reactions.

As already mentioned, the ionization of a gas provides a means of detecting radiation and the first widely used radiation unit, the **roentgen**, was based on the ionizing effect on air of X and γ radiation. This unit had several limitations and so two further units, the **rad** and the **rem**, were introduced. Later, these two units were replaced in the SI system (Système International d'Unités) by the **gray** and the **sievert**, respectively.

The **gray** and the **sievert** have been approved by the International Commission on Radiation Units and Measurements (ICRU) and used by the International Commission on Radiological Protection (ICRP). However, the older units, the rad and the rem, are still used in some countries and an explanation of the relationships between the old units and the SI units is given in Appendix A.

3.3 ABSORBED DOSE

Absorbed dose is a measure of energy deposition in any medium by any type of ionizing radiation. The original unit of absorbed dose was the rad, which was defined as an energy deposition of 0.01 J/kg.

The unit of absorbed dose in SI units is called the **gray (Gy)** and is defined as an energy deposition of 1 J/kg. Thus:

$$1 \text{ Gy} = 1 \text{ J/kg}$$

When quoting an absorbed dose, it is important to specify the absorbing medium.

3.4 EQUIVALENT DOSE

Although the quantity **absorbed dose** is a very useful physical concept, it transpires that in biological systems the same degree of damage is not necessarily produced by the same absorbed dose of different types of radiation. It is found, for example, that 0.05 Gy of fast neutrons can do as much biological damage as 1 Gy of γ radiation. This difference in the radiobiological effectiveness must be taken into account if we wish to add doses of different radiations to obtain the total biologically effective dose. To do this we must multiply the absorbed dose of each type of radiation by a **radiation weighting factor (w_R)** which reflects the ability of the particular type of radiation to cause damage. The quantity obtained when absorbed dose is multiplied by w_R is known as **equivalent dose.**

The unit of equivalent dose in SI units is the **sievert (Sv)**, which is related to the gray as follows:

$$\text{equivalent dose (Sv)} = \text{absorbed dose (Gy)} \times w_R$$

The value of the radiation weighting factor is found to depend on the density of ionization caused by the radiation. An α particle produces about 10^6 ion pairs per millimetre of track in tissue whereas a β particle produces about 10 000/mm. The factor, w_R, is assigned a value of one for γ radiation and the values for other types of radiation are related to this in accordance with their ionization densities. Beta radiation causes ionization of a similar density to γ radiation and so the weighting factor is also one for β radiation. The value of w_R for neutrons depends on the neutron energy and varies from five for thermal neutrons to 20 for fast. For α and other multiply-charged particles w_R is also taken as 20. The values of w_R for the most commonly encountered radiations are summarized in Table 3.1.

Table 3.1 Summary of values of w_R

Type of radiation	w_R
X-rays, γ-rays and electrons	1
Protons	5
Thermal neutrons	5
Fast neutrons	5–20*
Alpha particles, fission fragments	20

*Depending on energy

> ### EXAMPLE 3.1
>
> In 1 year a worker receives a gamma dose of 0.01 Gy, a thermal neutron (N_s) dose of 0.001 Gy, and a fast neutron dose (N_f) of 0.0002 Gy. What is his total equivalent dose? (Take w_R for fast neutrons as 20.)
>
> | | | |
> |---|---|---|
> | Equivalent dose | = absorbed dose × radiation weighting factor | |
> | Equivalent dose, γ | = 0.01 × 1 | = 0.01 Sv |
> | Equivalent dose, N_s | = 0.001 × 5 | = 0.005 Sv |
> | Equivalent dose, N_f | = 0.0002 × 20 | = 0.004 Sv |
> | | | |
> | Total equivalent dose | | = 0.019 Sv |

In the remainder of the book, we generally refer to **equivalent dose** simply as dose, except where this could lead to confusion.

3.5 EFFECTIVE DOSE

A further complication is that different organs and tissues have differing sensitivities to radiation and, to deal with the very common situation in which the body is not uniformly exposed, another concept is needed and this is called **effective dose**, E. This is obtained by summing the equivalent doses to all tissues and organs of the body, multiplied by a weighting factor w_T for each tissue or organ. This is written:

$$E = \sum_T H_T w_T$$

where H_T is the equivalent dose in tissue T. The basis of the organ weighting factors is discussed further in Chapters 4 and 7. It should be noted that effective dose also uses units of sieverts (Sv).

3.6 SUBMULTIPLES

In terms of the levels of radiation exposure encountered in the working environment, the gray and the sievert are very large units. It is often convenient to have smaller units and this is done by using the prefixes **milli** (one-thousandth) abbreviated to m, and **micro** (one-millionth) abbreviated to μ. Thus:

$$1 \text{ Gy} = 1000 \text{ mGy} = 1\,000\,000 \text{ } \mu\text{Gy}$$

$$1 \text{ Sv} = 1000 \text{ mSv} = 1\,000\,000 \text{ } \mu\text{Sv}$$

EXAMPLE 3.2

On three successive days a nuclear reactor operator received the following doses of gamma radiation:

Day 1   95 μSv

Day 2   5 μSv

Day 3   1 mSv

What was his total dose in mSv over the three days?

Day	Dose	mSv
1	$95\,\mu Sv = \dfrac{95}{1000}\,mSv$	0.095
2	$5\,\mu Sv = \dfrac{5}{1000}\,mSv$	0.005
3	$1\,mSv$	1.000
	Total dose =	1.100 mSv

3.7 DOSE RATE

The gray and sievert are units expressing an amount of radiation that may have been received over any period of time. In controlling the radiation hazard it is usually necessary to know the rate at which the radiation is being received. The relationship between dose, dose rate and time is:

$$\text{dose} = \text{dose rate} \times \text{time}$$

Thus if someone works in an area for 2 h and receives a dose of 4 mSv, then the **dose rate** in that area is 2 mSv/h. Similarly, **absorbed dose rates** are expressed in Gy/h.

EXAMPLE 3.3

If a man is permitted to receive a total dose of 1 mSv in a week, for how many hours may he work in an area in which the dose rate is 50 μSv/h?

$$\text{Dose} = \text{dose rate} \times \text{time}$$

$$\text{Time} = \frac{1\,mSv}{50\,\mu Sv/h} = \frac{1000\,\mu Sv}{50\,\mu Sv/h} = 20\ h$$

3.8 FLUX

It is often convenient to express a radiation field as the number of particles or photons crossing an area of 1 square metre in 1 second. This is strictly **fluence rate**, but is commonly referred to as **flux** (denoted by Φ). The concept is best illustrated by a practical example.

Consider a point source which emits neutrons at the rate of Q per second (Fig. 3.3). The flux at distance r is the number of neutrons passing through an area of $1\,m^2$ per second. Since the neutrons are being emitted uniformly in all directions, the flux at distance r is the number of neutrons emitted per second divided by the area of the sphere of radius r. This area is $4\pi r^2$ and so the flux Φ is given by:

$$\Phi = \frac{Q}{4\pi r^2} \quad \text{neutrons per square metre per second } (n/(m^2 s))$$

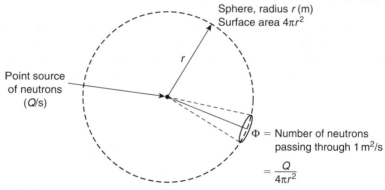

FIGURE 3.3 Flux from a point source.

Note that if r is doubled, r^2 increases fourfold and Φ reduces by four times. This relationship is the **inverse square law** which will be dealt with in greater detail in Chapter 8.

EXAMPLE 3.4

Calculate the flux at a distance of 0.5 m from a source which emits 2×10^7 n/s.

$$\Phi = \frac{Q}{4\pi r^2}$$

$$= \frac{2 \times 10^7}{4\pi \times 0.5 \times 0.5}$$

$$= 6.4 \times 10^6 \text{ n/m}^2\text{s}.$$

EXAMPLE 3.5

Calculate the gamma photon flux at 1 m from a 0.1 TBq cobalt-60 source. (Cobalt-60 emits two γ-rays per disintegration.) From Chapter 2, we know that 0.1 TBq $= 10^{11}$ dis/s, but for ^{60}Co there are two γ-photons per disintegration. Therefore:

$$Q = 2 \times 10^{11} \text{ photons/s}$$

$$\Phi = \frac{Q}{4\pi r^2}$$

$$= \frac{2 \times 10^{11}}{4\pi \times 1^2}$$

$$= 1.6 \times 10^{10} \ \gamma \text{ photons/(m}^2\text{s).}$$

3.9 RELATIONSHIP OF UNITS

The relationship of the units which have now been introduced is illustrated in Fig. 3.4. The gray describes an absorbed dose in any medium and the sievert expresses biological effect on the human body. In health physics, it is clearly the biological effect of radiation that is of interest and so whenever possible equivalent dose or effective dose should be used.

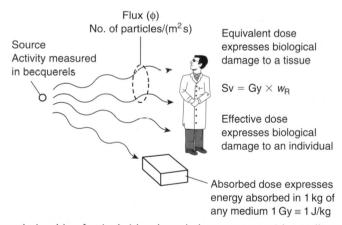

Flux (ϕ)
No. of particles/(m^{2}s)

Source
Activity measured
in becquerels

Equivalent dose
expresses biological
damage to a tissue

$Sv = Gy \times w_R$

Effective dose
expresses biological
damage to an individual

Absorbed dose expresses
energy absorbed in 1 kg of
any medium 1 Gy $\equiv$ 1 J/kg

FIGURE 3.4 The relationship of units (with acknowledgements to Lt Cdr J. Kelly, RN).

In everyday health physics, the term **dose** is often loosely used to mean either of the quantities **absorbed dose** or **equivalent dose**. In the following chapters the term **dose** will generally be taken to mean either **equivalent dose** or **effective dose** depending on the context.

SUMMARY OF CHAPTER

Radiation: transfers energy from the source to the absorbing medium.
Ionization: removal of orbital electron – production of ion pairs.

Ionization chamber: application of electric field causes a current of ions to flow.

Absorbed dose: energy deposition in any medium by any type of ionizing radiation. $1\,\mathrm{Gy} = 1\,\mathrm{J/kg}$.

Equivalent dose: measure of the biological effect of radiation, the unit is the sievert.

$$\text{Equivalent dose} = \text{absorbed dose} \times \text{radiation weighting factor.}$$

Radiation weighting factor, w_R: measure of the ability of a particular type of radiation to cause biological damage, related to the density of ionization. $w_R = 1$ for β, X and γ, 5 for protons and thermal neutrons, 5–20 for fast neutrons and 20 for α particles.

Effective dose: an indicator of the effects of radiation on the body as a whole when different body tissues are exposed to different levels of equivalent dose.

Tissue weighting factor, w_T: a factor reflecting the radiosensitivity of a particular tissue or organ.

Dose = dose rate $\times$ time.

Flux from point source = $Q/4\pi r^2$.

REVISION QUESTIONS

1. What is ionization and how can it be used as a means of measuring radiation?
2. What is a **gray**?
3. Explain why the **sievert** is a more suitable unit in health physics than the **gray**.
4. Explain the concepts of **equivalent dose** and **effective dose**.
5. Calculate the neutron flux at a distance of 0.3 m from a neutron source which emits 3×10^7 neutrons per second.
6. In 1 week an operator on a nuclear reactor works for 4 h in an area in which the γ and neutron dose rates respectively are 5 μSv/h and 7 μSv/h, and for a further 18 h in an area in which the γ dose rate is 2 μSv/h (no neutrons). Calculate his dose for the week.
7. A worker receives an external dose in 1 year of 1 mSv (assumed to be uniform over the whole body). In addition, as a result of an intake of radioactivity, an equivalent dose of 4 mSv is delivered to the thyroid, for which the organ weighting factor is 0.05. What is his effective dose for the year?

Biological effects of radiation   ■ 4

4.1 INTRODUCTION

The interaction of ionizing radiation with the human body, arising either from **external** sources outside the body or from **internal** contamination of the body by radioactive substances, leads to biological effects which may later show up as clinical symptoms. The nature and severity of these symptoms and the time at which they appear depend on the amount of radiation absorbed and the rate at which it is received. In addition to the effects on the person receiving the dose, damage to the germ cells in the reproductive organs – the gonads – can result in hereditary effects which arise in later generations.

4.2 BASIC HUMAN PHYSIOLOGY

Physiology is concerned with the functions of the body as a whole and the component organs and systems. Some basic knowledge of physiology is necessary for an understanding of the ways in which radioactivity can enter and become distributed in the body. Humans can be regarded as machines consisting of various interrelated systems, each performing some important function. The systems which are most relevant to an understanding of the behaviour of radioactive substances which enter the body are the circulatory, respiratory and digestive systems (see Fig. 4.1).

4.2.1 The circulatory system

The circulatory system is a closed circuit of tubes around which the blood is pumped by the action of the **heart**. Blood is the transport mechanism of the body and it circulates to almost every region carrying food and oxygen to the cells. It also picks up waste products and carbon dioxide and transfers them to the excretory organs. The heart is actually two pumps: the left side pumps the blood through the **arteries** to the tissues. Nourishment is transferred from the tissues to the cells via the tissue fluid. The blood, after passing through the tissues, returns to the right side of the heart via the **veins**. The blood is then pumped to the **lungs** where it becomes oxygenated before returning to the left side of the heart.

  The blood in the arteries contains a lot of oxygen and is bright red in colour while the blood returning from the tissues contains very little oxygen and is dark red. The body contains about 5 litres of blood which circulates about once a minute. There are three types of

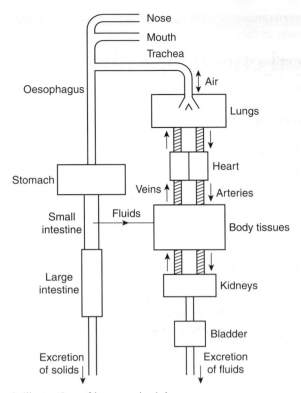

FIGURE 4.1 Schematic illustration of human physiology.

blood cells, each performing an essential function: **red cells** (erythrocytes), **white cells** (granulocytes and lymphocytes) and **platelets** (thrombocytes). The function of the red cells is to transport the food and oxygen required by the body, whereas the white cells serve as a means of defence against infection by digesting microorganisms. Platelets play a vital role in the formation of clots at the site of injuries.

4.2.2 The respiratory system

Respiration (or breathing) is the method by which oxygen is taken into the lungs and carbon dioxide eliminated. The oxygen is absorbed by the blood as it passes through the lungs and carried to the tissues as described above. The tissues produce carbon dioxide as a gaseous waste product and this is carried back by the blood to the lungs and breathed out. The volume of air breathed per day is approximately 20 m³, of which half is usually considered to be breathed during the 8 h of work.

In the process of respiration, airborne contaminants, either in the form of gaseous or particulate materials (i.e. airborne dusts) are inhaled. Gases pass freely into the lungs and enter the bloodstream to a greater or lesser extent, depending on their solubility. In the case of particulate matter, only a fraction of the inhaled material is deposited in the lungs, the remainder is either exhaled or deposited in the upper respiratory passages and subsequently swallowed. The behaviour of the material deposited in the lungs depends mainly on its solubility. Highly soluble materials are absorbed rapidly into the bloodstream, perhaps in a matter of hours, whereas insoluble material may persist in the lungs for many months. Clearly, then, the respiratory system represents a route of entry for radioactive substances which can remain in the lungs for long periods or be transported by the blood-stream to other parts of the body.

4.2.3 The digestive system

The digestive system consists of the oesophagus, the stomach, the duodenum and the small intestine, which is connected to the large intestine. Food taken in by the mouth is converted into a form suitable for the production of heat and energy, and the molecules necessary for the growth and repair of tissues. The large molecules in the food are broken down by enzymes in the digestive tract before being absorbed into the bloodstream and passed via the liver to the tissues. The unabsorbed food, together with bacteria and cells shed from the intestine wall, is passed out as solid waste (faeces). Liquid waste (the waste products of cells dissolved in water) is excreted from the body via the kidneys and bladder as urine.

Soluble radioactive contamination, when swallowed, may pass through the walls of the digestive tract and become absorbed into the bloodstream, which carries it to all parts of the body. It is then likely to become concentrated mainly in some specific organ or tissue, which it will irradiate until it decays or is excreted. Insoluble contamination passes through the digestive tract and is excreted in the faeces. During its passage through the body it will irradiate the tract and the large intestine.

4.3 CELL BIOLOGY

All living creatures and organisms consist of tiny structures known as cells. The basic components of a cell are the **nucleus**, a surrounding liquid known as the **cytoplasm** and a **membrane** which forms the cell wall. Figure 4.2 shows a simplified representation of a 'typical' human cell.

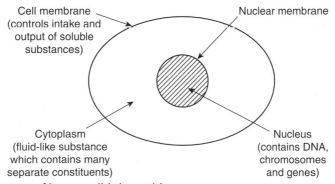

FIGURE 4.2 Structure of human cell (schematic).

The simplest picture of the cell is that the cytoplasm is the 'factory' of the cell while the nucleus contains all the information which the cell needs to carry out its function and reproduce itself. The cytoplasm breaks down food and converts it into energy and small molecules. These small molecules are later converted into complex molecules needed by the cell either for maintenance or duplication.

The nucleus contains chromosomes, which are tiny threadlike structures made up of genes. Human cells normally contain 46 chromosomes. The genes consist of deoxyribonucleic acid (DNA) and protein molecules, and carry the information which determines the characteristics of the daughter cell.

Cells are able to reproduce to compensate for cells that die. The life of different types of human cell, and hence the rate of reproduction, varies from a few hours to many years. Reproduction of cells occurs in two ways, known as **mitosis** and **meiosis**. The mitotic cells are the ordinary cells in the body and in mitosis the chromosomes duplicate by splitting length-ways. The original cell then divides into two new cells, each identical to the original cell.

Meiosis is a special kind of division which occurs during the formation of the sexual reproduction cells, namely the sperm in the male and the ovum in the female. It occurs only once in the cell's life-cycle and only in the reproductive cells. In sexual reproduction a sperm and an ovum unite and the chromosomes combine to form a new cell containing genetic material (i.e. genes) from each of the parents. The embryo and subsequently the offspring develops from this single cell (the fertilized ovum).

4.4 THE INTERACTION OF RADIATION WITH CELLS

The basic difference between nuclear radiations and the more commonly encountered radiations such as heat and light is that the former have sufficient energy to cause ioniza-tion. In water, of which cells are largely composed, ionization can lead to molecular changes and to the formation of chemical species of a type that is damaging to the chromo-some material. The damage takes the form of changes in the construction and function of the cell. In the human body, these changes may manifest themselves as clinical symptoms such as radiation sickness, cataracts or, in the longer term, cancer.

This overall process is usually considered to occur in four stages, as follows:

1. **The initial physical stage**, lasting only an extremely small fraction ($c.~10^{-16}$) of a second in which energy is deposited in the cell and causes ionization. In water the process may be written as:

$$H_2O \xrightarrow{\text{radiation}} H_2O^+ + e^-$$

   where H_2O^+ is the positive ion and e^- is the negative ion.

2. **The physicochemical stage**, lasting about 10^{-6} s, in which the ions interact with other water molecules resulting in a number of new products. For example, the posi-tive ion dissociates:

$$H_2O^+ \longrightarrow H^+ + OH$$

   The negative ion, that is the electron, attaches to a neutral water molecule which then dissociates:

$$H_2O + e^- \longrightarrow H_2O^-$$

$$H_2O^- \longrightarrow H + OH^-$$

Thus the products of the reactions are H^+, OH^-, H and OH. The first two ions, which are present to quite a large extent in ordinary water, take no part in subsequent reactions. The other two products, H and OH, are called **free radicals**, that is, they have an unpaired electron and are chemically highly reactive. Another reaction product is hydrogen peroxide, H_2O_2, which is a strong oxidizing agent and is formed by the reaction:

$$OH + OH \longrightarrow H_2O_2$$

3. **The chemical stage**, lasting a few seconds, in which the reaction products interact with the important organic molecules of the cell. The free radicals and oxidizing agents may attack the complex molecules which form the chromosomes. They may, for example, attach themselves to a molecule or cause links in long chain molecules to be broken.
4. **The biological stage**, in which the time scale varies from tens of minutes to tens of years depending on the particular symptoms. The chemical changes discussed above can affect an individual cell in a number of ways. For example, they may result in:
   (a) the early death of the cell or the prevention or delay of cell division; or
   (b) a permanent modification which is passed on to daughter cells.

The effects of radiation on the human body as a whole arise from damage to individual cells, but the two types of change have quite different results.

In the first case, the death or prevention of division of cells results in the depletion of the cell population within organs of the body. Below a certain level of dose (a threshold), the proportion of cells damaged will not be sufficient to affect the function of the organ and there will be no observable effect on the organ or the body as a whole. Above the threshold, effects will start to be observed and the severity of the effects will increase quite rapidly as the dose increases. This type of effect is referred to as **deterministic**. This means that within the range of variability between individuals, the relationship between the dose and the severity of the effects can be assessed with reasonable confidence.

In the second case, modification of even a single cell may result, after a latency period, in a cancer in the exposed individual or, if the modification is to a reproductive cell, the damage may be transmitted to later generations and give rise to **hereditary** effects. In these cases, it is the likelihood of the effect occurring that depends on the dose. This type of effect is referred to as **stochastic**, meaning 'of a random or statistical nature'.

To summarize, radiation-induced changes at the cellular level can lead to two distinct types of injury.

1. **Deterministic effects** in which, above a certain threshold dose, the severity of the effects increase with increasing dose. These effects are discussed in Section 4.5.
2. **Stochastic effects**, in which the probability of occurrence of the effect increases with dose. The effects include cancer induction (see Section 4.6) and hereditary effects in future generations (see Section 4.7).

4.5 DETERMINISTIC EFFECTS

4.5.1 Acute radiation effects

The acute radiation effects are those that occur within a few weeks after the receipt of a large dose in a relatively short period of time. The effects result from a major depletion of cell populations in a number of body organs caused by cell-killing and the prevention or delay of cell division. The main effects are attributable to bone marrow, gastrointestinal or neuromuscular damage, depending on the dose received. Acute absorbed doses above about 1 Gy give rise to nausea and vomiting. This is known as radiation sickness and it occurs a few hours after exposure as a result of damage to cells lining the intestine. Absorbed doses above about 2 Gy can lead to death, probably 10–15 days after exposures.

There is no well-defined threshold dose below which there is no risk of death from acute doses, although below about 1.5 Gy the risk of early death would be very low. Similarly, there is no well-defined point above which death is certain, but the chances of surviving an acute dose of about 8 Gy would be very low. A reasonable estimate can be made of the dose which would be lethal for 50 per cent of the exposed subjects within 60 days of exposure. This is called LD_{50}^{60} and is thought to have a value of between 3 Gy and 5 Gy for man. For doses up to about 10 Gy, death is usually caused by secondary infections that result from depletion of the white blood cells that normally provide protection against infection. The range of doses from 3 to 10 Gy is often called the region of **infection death**. In this range the chances of survival can be increased by special medical treatments, which include isolating the subject in a sterile (i.e. infection-free) environment and giving bone marrow transfusion to stimulate white blood cell production.

For doses above about 10 Gy survival time drops abruptly to between 3 days and 5 days. It remains at about this figure until much higher doses are reached. In this region the radiation dose causes severe depletion of the cells lining the intestine. Gross damage occurs in the lining of the intestine, followed by severe bacterial invasion. This is called the region of **gastrointestinal death**.

At much higher doses, survival times become progressively shorter. There are very few human data in this region but, from animal experiments, the symptoms indicate some damage to the central nervous system; hence, the region is called the region of **central nervous system death**. However, it is found that death is not instantaneous even in animals irradiated with doses in excess of 500 Gy.

Another effect which shows up soon after an acute over-exposure to radiation is **erythema**, that is, reddening of the skin. In many situations the skin is subject to more radiation exposure than most other tissues. This is especially true for β-rays and low-energy X-rays. A dose of about 3 Gy of low-energy X-rays will result in erythema and larger exposures may lead to other symptoms such as changes in pigmentation, blistering and ulceration.

The levels of exposure of workers and members of the public arising from normal operations in the nuclear energy industry, or from industrial and medical applications of radiation, are far below the levels that would induce early effects. Such high doses could only be received in the unlikely event of an accident. However, the low doses received in normal operations may cause harmful effects in the long term and these are discussed below.

It will have been noted that in this discussion, early effects have been considered in terms of the absorbed dose, expressed in gray (Gy), rather than as equivalent dose in sievert (Sv). This is really a question of definition; the radiation weighting factor, w_R, discussed in the previous chapter, and hence the concept of equivalent dose, is intended to apply only to exposures within the normal recommended limits (see Chapter 6) and should not be applied to doses at levels which could lead to early effects.

4.5.2 Late deterministic effects

Another radiation effect which is deterministic in nature but which may not occur for many years is damage to the lens of the eye. This takes the form of observable opacities in the lens or, in extreme cases, visual impairment as the result of a cataract. Again, there is a threshold dose and so, by setting a dose limit for the lens of the eye, the occurrence of these effects can be prevented (see Chapter 6).

There is some evidence from animal experiments that exposure to radiation may slightly reduce the life expectation of individuals who do not exhibit any specific radiation-induced symptoms. Observations of human populations exposed at relatively high levels indicate that, if life-shortening occurs at all, it is very slight, almost certainly less than 1 year per sievert.

4.6 STOCHASTIC EFFECTS – CANCER INDUCTION

It became apparent in the early part of the twentieth century that groups of people such as radiologists and their patients, who were exposed to relatively high levels of radiation, showed a higher incidence of certain types of cancer than groups not exposed to radiation. More recently, detailed studies of the populations exposed to radiation from atomic bombs, of patients exposed to radiation therapy and of groups exposed occupationally, particularly uranium miners, have confirmed the ability of radiation to induce cancer.

Cancer is an over-proliferation of cells in a body organ. It is thought that cancer may result from damage to the control system of a single cell, causing it to divide more rapidly than a normal cell. The defect is transmitted to the daughter cells so the population of abnormal cells builds up to the detriment of the normal cells in the organ. The estimation of the increased risk of cancer is complicated by the long and variable latent period, from about 5 to 30 years or more, between exposure and the appearance of the cancer, and by the fact that radiation-induced cancers are not normally distinguishable from those that arise spontaneously. The incidence of cancer in a normal population is high, with about one person in three expected to die eventually from some form of cancer. This high background makes it very difficult to establish whether any additional cases of a particular type of cancer are the result of radiation exposure, even in populations that have been exposed at relatively high levels.

At the high doses and dose rates experienced by the groups mentioned earlier, the International Commission on Radiological Protection (ICRP; see Chapter 6) has estimated that, averaged over a typical population of all ages, a dose of 1 Sv to each individual would result in a radiation-induced fatal cancer in about 10 per cent of the persons exposed. This is the same as saying that the average risk to an individual from a dose of 1 Sv is about one in 10 or 0.1. The extrapolation of this estimate to the much lower doses and dose rates normally encountered as a result of operations in the nuclear industry and elsewhere introduces further uncertainty. A very conservative approach would be to make a linear extrapolation from high to low dose. Since a dose of 1 Sv carries a risk of fatal cancer of 0.1, the risk from a dose of 1 mSv would be 1000 times lower, or 0.0001. However, on the basis of theoretical considerations, experiments on animals and other organisms, and limited human data, ICRP concluded that this is likely to overestimate the risks of radiation exposure at low doses and dose rates by a factor of between two and ten. This factor is referred to as the **Dose and Dose Rate Effectiveness Factor (DDREF)** and, to err on the safe side, ICRP recommends using only the factor of two. This means that the additional risk of fatal cancer imposed on an average individual by exposure to radiation at low doses and dose rates can be estimated using a **dose – risk factor** of 0.05 per sievert (this is usually written as $5 \times 10^{-2}\,\text{Sv}^{-1}$). Using this factor, the risk of fatal cancer due to a given dose can be estimated using the relationship:

$$\text{Risk} = \text{Dose (Sv)} \times \text{risk factor (Sv}^{-1})$$

For a dose of 10 mSv (0.01 Sv), the risk of fatal cancer would be:

$$\text{Risk} = 0.01\,\text{Sv} \times 5 \times 10^{-2}\,\text{Sv}^{-1} = 5 \times 10^{-4}$$

In addition to fatal cancers, exposure to radiation also gives rise to cancers which are non-fatal or curable. These need to be taken into account but it would clearly be inappropriate to give them the same weight as fatal cancers. Recognizing this, ICRP has developed the concept of **detriment** that allows effects of different importance to be combined to give an overall measure of the detrimental effects of radiation exposure. This is discussed further in Section 4.8.

4.7 STOCHASTIC EFFECTS – HEREDITARY

The hereditary effects of radiation result from damage to the reproductive cells. This damage takes the form of alterations, known as **genetic mutations**, in the hereditary material of the cell.

It has already been mentioned that reproduction occurs when the ovum is fertilized by a sperm. As a result, the offspring receives a complete set of genetic material from each parent. Thus the child receives two complementary sets of genes, one from each of its parents. In general it is found that one gene is 'dominant' and the other 'recessive'. The dominant gene determines the particular characteristic with which it is associated.

Recessive genes are only recognized when, by chance, two of the recessive-type genes come together. A considerable number of diseases are associated with recessive genes and will therefore only manifest themselves when both parents have the same recessive genes. Spontaneous mutation accounts for the fact that an appreciable fraction of the world's population suffers from one of the 500 or more defects or diseases attributable to hereditary effects.

Radiation can induce gene mutations which are indistinguishable from naturally occurring mutations. It should be noted in passing that heat and chemicals can also cause mutations. Mutated genes can be either dominant, in which case their effects would manifest themselves in the first generation of offspring, or recessive, when the effect would not occur in the first generation. A recessive mutation will only result in an effect if the same mutation is inherited from both parents. It is generally assumed that all mutations are harmful, although this cannot be strictly true since man has attained his present advanced state via a series of mutations. However, this has occurred over an immense time-span and the number of harmful mutations which have had to be eliminated from the species over this time is incalculably large.

Since ionizing radiation can cause an increase in the mutation rate, its use will increase the number of genetically abnormal people present in future generations. Clearly, the consequences of excessive genetic damage would be very serious indeed and strict control must be exercised over the radiation exposure of the general population.

The risks of hereditary effects due to exposure of the gonads are very uncertain. The ICRP estimates the risk of serious hereditary health effects in all generations following the irradiation of either parent at low doses and dose rates to be about 3×10^{-2} per sievert, averaged over the whole population. Clearly, only that exposure which occurs up to the time of conception can affect the genetic characteristics of the offspring and, since the mean age of childbearing is about 30 years, only a proportion of the dose received by a typical population will be genetically harmful. The total genetic risk in all generations, averaged over both sexes and all ages, is therefore about 1.3×10^{-2} per sievert. In a population of working age, because of the different age distribution, the risk is about 0.8×10^{-2} per sievert.

4.8 DETRIMENT

To assist in quantifying and combining the consequences of exposure of different organs and tissues of the body, the ICRP has developed the concept of **detriment**. This takes into account the relative risks and the average latent period of fatal cancers in different organs, an allowance for the ill-health resulting from non-fatal cancers and an allowance for the risk of serious hereditary effects in all future generations descended from an exposed individual. Table 4.1 shows the contributions of the main organs of the body to the detriment. The second column shows the probability of fatal cancer in each organ for an equivalent dose to that organ of 1 Sv. The third column gives the probability of severe genetic effects in future generations from an equivalent dose of 1 Sv to the gonads. The final column shows the relative contribution of each organ to the overall detriment, taking account of the factors discussed above.

These estimates of the relative contributions to the overall detriment from radiation exposure provide the basis for definition of the **tissue weighting factors**, w_T, used to calculate the quantity **effective dose**, as discussed in Chapter 3 and further explained in Chapter 6.

Table 4.1 Relative contribution of organs to total detriment

Organ or tissue	Probability of fatal cancer, $10^{-4}\,\mathrm{Sv}^{-1}$	Probability of serious genetic effects, $10^{-4}\,\mathrm{Sv}^{-1}$	Relative contribution to detriment
Bladder	30		0.040
Bone marrow	50		0.143
Bone surface	5		0.009
Breast	20		0.050
Colon	85		0.141
Liver	15		0.022
Lung	85		0.111
Oesophagus	30		0.034
Ovary	10		0.020
Skin	2		0.006
Stomach	110		0.139
Thyroid	8		0.021
Remainder	50		0.081
Gonads		100	0.183
Total	500	100	1.00

SUMMARY OF CHAPTER

Physiology: the study of the functions of the body as a whole and its component organs and systems.
Heart: pumps blood to all parts of the body via the arteries and the veins.
Blood: carries food and oxygen to cells and removes waste products.
Red blood cells: transport food and oxygen.

White blood cells: defend the body against infection.

Platelets: vital to the formation of clots.

Respiration: method by which oxygen is taken into the lungs and carbon dioxide eliminated.

Digestive system: converts food into a form suitable for the production of heat and energy, and molecules necessary for the growth and repair of tissues.

Stages in radiation damage process:

1. Initial physical stage ($c.\ 10^{-16}$ s) consisting of ionization and excitation of atoms and molecules.
2. Physicochemical stage (10^{-8}–10^{-5} s) consisting of dissociation of ions and formation of free radicals.
3. Chemical stage (a few seconds) consisting of the interaction of free radicals with other molecules in the body.
4. Biological stage (minutes to years) in which the chemical reactions show up as effects in individual cells.

Components of cell: nucleus, cytoplasm and outer membrane.

Nucleus: contains chromosomes which are threadlike structures made up of genes.

Genes: carry the information which determines the characteristics of daughter cells.

Mitosis: process by which single cells reproduce.

Meiosis: a stage in the formation of the reproductive cells – the sperm in the male and the ovum in the female.

Effects of radiation on cells: inhibition of mitosis, chromosome aberrations.

Acute effects: effects occurring within a few weeks of a very large exposure; due to depletion of cell populations.

Late effects: effects occurring at later times, typically some years after exposure; main effect is cancer induction.

Hereditary effects: may appear in descendants of exposed individuals.

Stochastic effects: probability of occurrence depends on dose; mainly cancer and genetic effects.

Deterministic effects: severity depends on dose; mainly the early radiation effects plus certain late effects, such as cataract formation.

REVISION QUESTIONS

1. Describe how radioactivity can be deposited in various organs of the body: (a) if it is inhaled, and (b) if it is ingested (swallowed).
2. List the four stages in the radiation damage process.
3. Distinguish between deterministic and stochastic effects of radiation.
4. What are the acute radiation effects? Discuss the severity of the effects over the dose range 1–10 Gy.
5. What is the major late effect of radiation and upon what assumptions are risk estimates based?

Natural and man-made radiation   5

5.1 INTRODUCTION

Throughout history man has been exposed to radiation from the environment. This natural background radiation comes from three main sources: cosmic radiation, radiation from terrestrial sources and radioactivity in the body.

It is impossible to decide whether the natural background radiation has been harmful or beneficial to the development of the human species. It was pointed out in the previous chapter that a very small, but finite, fraction of the natural mutations in cells must be beneficial since they have contributed to the evolution of higher forms of life. Conversely, some genetic mutations lead to hereditary defects and genetic death. It is clear that these two effects have achieved some sort of balance and that life has evolved to its present state despite background radiation, or perhaps even because of it.

In addition to the natural sources of background radiation many artificial sources of radiation have been introduced since the discovery of X-rays and radioactivity at the end of the nineteenth century, and particularly since the exploitation of the process of nuclear fission in the middle of the twentieth century. These artificial sources now add a significant contribution to the total radiation exposure of the population.

5.2 COSMIC RADIATION

Cosmic radiation reaches the Earth from interstellar space and from the Sun. It is composed of a very wide range of penetrating radiations which undergo many types of reactions with the elements they encounter in the atmosphere. The atmosphere acts as a shield and reduces very considerably the amount of cosmic radiation reaching the Earth's surface. This filtering action means that the dose rate at sea-level is less than at high altitudes. For example, the mean dose rate from cosmic radiation at sea-level, at the equator, is about 0.2 mSv/year, while the dose rate at an altitude of 3000 m is about 1 mSv/year. The average dose rate in the British Isles from cosmic radiation is about 0.33 mSv/year.

One very important radionuclide arises mainly from the interaction of neutrons in cosmic radiation with nitrogen in the upper atmosphere to form carbon-14 as follows:

$$^{14}N(n, p)^{14}C$$

Carbon-14, which has a half-life of 5568 years, diffuses to the lower atmosphere where it may become incorporated in living matter. Similarly, small concentrations of other radionuclides such as tritium (^{3}H, half-life 12.26 years), chlorine-36 (^{36}Cl, half-life 3.08×10^5 years) and calcium-41 (^{41}Ca, half-life 1.1×10^5 years) are maintained in the lower atmosphere by cosmic ray reactions. They are much less important than ^{14}C.

5.3 RADIATION FROM TERRESTRIAL SOURCES

The rocks and soil of the Earth's strata contain small quantities of the radioactive elements uranium and thorium with their daughter products. The concentration of these elements varies considerably depending on the type of rock formation. In sandstone and limestone regions the concentration is much lower than in granite. Thus the dose rate depends on the geographic location. In the British Isles, the average effective dose of γ radiation from this source is about 0.35 mSv/year. In some areas, the dose rate may be several times higher than this value.

Other long-lived isotopes such as ^{48}Ca (half-life $> 7 \times 10^8$ years) and ^{50}V (half-life 4×10^{14} years) occur naturally but in very low concentrations and do not contribute significantly to human dose.

5.4 NATURALLY OCCURRING RADIOACTIVE MATERIAL (NORM)

The presence of naturally occurring radioactivity in rocks and soil also means that most natural materials are slightly radioactive. Usually, the resulting radiation exposure is trivial but there are materials that can cause significant exposure, either because they contain higher levels of naturally occurring radioactivity or because they are processed or used in such a way as to enhance the exposure. These materials are known as NORM (naturally occurring radioactive materials). Where materials are processed, the concentrations of the radioactivity can be increased in some of the process streams and give rise to exposure of workers in the processing plant. In other cases the products of processing, such as consumer products or building materials, can contain enhanced levels of activity and result in increased radiation exposure of the general population.

In the oil and gas industries, naturally occurring radium and its daughter products can build up as scale in pipes and vessels. The descaling of these results in occupational radiation exposure and in waste streams containing radium. In the smelting of iron ore, high concentrations of lead-210 and polonium-210 occur in dusts and residues. In other metal smelting applications, the use of special mineral sands containing natural uranium and thorium can lead to exposures either directly or from the enhanced concentrations in foundry slag. Another material containing levels of uranium, thorium and potassium that can be of radiological significance is phosphate rock. This is often used as an agricultural fertilizer. In addition, gypsum, which arises as a byproduct of phosphate processing, is widely used in building materials.

It is the responsibility of enterprises that extract, process or use NORM to establish by appropriate surveys and assessments whether the doses from NORM are likely to be of radiological significance and, where necessary, introduce adequate measures to ensure that exposures are kept as low as reasonably practicable.

5.5 RADIOACTIVITY IN THE BODY

The ingestion and inhalation of naturally occurring radionuclides gives rise to a dose which varies considerably depending on the location, diet and habits of the individual concerned. Potassium-40 and nuclides from the uranium and thorium series contribute most to this dose, with a minor contribution from carbon-14, which is produced by the interaction of cosmic particles with stable carbon, nitrogen and oxygen in the atmosphere.

A significant contribution to the radioactivity in the body comes from the gaseous decay products of the uranium and thorium radioactive series, namely radon and thoron. These gases diffuse from the rocks and soil and are present in easily measurable concentrations in the atmosphere. In the open air their concentrations, and hence their radiological impact, are low. However, within buildings high concentrations can occur because of diffusion of the gases from building materials or from the ground, and because of restricted ventilation. The radioactive daughter products of radon and thoron attach themselves to dust particles in the air and when these are inhaled they result in radiation exposure, particularly of the lungs.

The average annual dose to members of the UK population from this source is about 1.3 mSv/year, but recent studies have shown that in some dwellings the dose rate can be up to 100 times the average. As a result, there are programmes in a number of countries to identify dwellings and places of work having high concentrations and, where necessary, to undertake remedial work. The approach used is to reduce ingress of the gases by sealing walls and floors, and to increase the ventilation.

Naturally occurring radioactivity is also taken up by plants and animals with the result that most foodstuffs contain measurable amounts of natural radioactivity. Of ordinary foods, cereals have a high radioactive content while milk produce, fruit and vegetables have a low content. The intake of natural radioactivity varies greatly with diet and with location. The average dose in the UK from this source is about 0.25 mSv/year.

5.6 SUMMARY OF DOSES FROM NATURAL RADIATION

Table 5.1 gives a list of typical average annual doses from natural radiation in the British Isles.

Table 5.1 Typical average annual doses from natural radiation

Source	Dose (mSv/year)
Local γ radiation	0.35
Radon, thoron and decay products	1.30
Cosmic radiation	0.33
Ingestion of natural radioactivity	0.25
Total	~2.20

Local gamma radiation comes from the ^{238}U and ^{232}Th series, and from ^{40}K. In certain parts of the world it is much higher than the value given in Table 5.1. For example, in the monazite sand regions of India and Brazil the annual whole-body doses from local γ radiation can be as much as 120 mSv/year.

5.7 MAN-MADE SOURCES OF RADIATION

The early experiences of man-made sources of radiation involved X-rays and various uses of radium. As early as 1896 a letter appeared in *Nature* describing the effects of repeated exposure of the hands to X-rays and during the next 15 years many more cases were reported. These cases arose both from experiments with X-ray sets and also from their use in various treatments. By 1911 Hesse had studied the histories of 94 cases of tumours induced in man by X-rays, of which 50 cases were among radiologists.

These studies illustrated the early forms of damage produced by X-rays and gave some indication of the longer-term effects. For some types of damage, such as skin cancer, there is a latent period of between 10 years and 30 years and some radiologists observed malignant skin changes as late as 25 years after discontinuing fluoroscopic examinations. By 1922 it was estimated that more than 100 radiologists had died from radiation-induced cancer. Similarly, it has been estimated that the death rate from leukaemia among early radiologists was about nine times that among other physicians.

Other studies have shown that the average life-expectancy of the pioneer radiologists was reduced by approximately 2–3 years compared with physicians in general practice. Using results from animal experiments on the relationship between life-shortening and amount of irradiation, it is estimated that the total dose received by the average radiologist from 1935 to 1958 was a few gray. The results of these studies have been used by the International Commission on Radiological Protection (ICRP) in deriving the risk factors for irradiation of organs and tissues of the body (see Chapter 6).

Experience was also gained early in the twentieth century of the effect of internal dose from various nuclides such as radium (^{226}Ra, half-life 1622 years), mesothorium (^{228}Ra, half-life 5.8 years), radiothorium (^{228}Th, half-life 1.91 years) and their daughter products. Even earlier, it had been recognized that there was a remarkably high incidence of lung cancer among the miners in the Schneeberg cobalt mines of Saxony and the Joachimsthal pitchblende mines in Bohemia. Eventually, this high rate of lung cancer was shown to be caused by radiation from the daughter products of uranium, namely ^{226}Ra, radon-222 (^{222}Rn), polonium-218 (^{218}Po) and others. These mines contain large concentrations of uranium.

During the second and third decades of the twentieth century there were many cases of over-exposure to radium. A considerable number of these arose from the use of radium as a therapeutic agent. It was administered for a large variety of diseases, ranging from arthritis to insanity.

The most serious over-exposures to radium occurred in the radium-dial painting industry in the USA. Most of the persons employed were women and they had the habit of 'pointing' their paint brushes with their lips. Many of these women probably ingested megabecquerel quantities of radium. Although the damaging effects of radium were eventually established, it is not known precisely how many radium-dial painters actually died from the effects of radiation damage. The study of people exposed to X-rays and radium is continuing to improve our estimates of the level of risk associated with acute and chronic exposures to radiation.

5.8 CURRENT SOURCES OF MAN-MADE RADIATION

In addition to the ever-present natural background radiation, there are several other sources of human exposure that have arisen only over the last 100 years or less. These are: diagnostic radiology, therapeutic radiology, use of isotopes in medicine, radioactive waste, fall-out from nuclear weapon tests, and occupational exposures to radiation.

5.8.1 Diagnostic radiology

It has been estimated that over 90 per cent of the total exposure of the population from medical uses of radiation comes from the diagnostic use of X-rays. The most important regions of the body in this context are the bone marrow, the gonads and the foetus. The bone marrow is the site of the primitive blood-forming cells and so irradiation of this region can lead to the induction of leukaemia. Irradiation of the gonads is important because of the possibility of genetic damage. Irradiation of pregnant women has to be controlled very strictly in order to limit the possibility of physical or mental damage to the child.

5.8.2 Therapeutic radiology

The average dose to the population from therapeutic radiology is less than that from diagnostic radiology. Although quite large exposures may be used in certain treatments, the number of people involved is much smaller.

5.8.3 Use of radioisotopes

Radioisotopes are used in medicine to give a means of tracing the path and location of specific chemicals in the body. Since radioactive isotopes are chemically identical to stable isotopes of the same element, they will follow the same path and be concentrated to the same degree as the non-active isotopes in the body. Using suitable detectors, the behaviour of the active, and hence by analogy of the ordinary non-active, isotopes of the element may be determined. At much higher concentrations, radioisotopes can be used for therapeutic purposes, see Chapter 13.

5.8.4 Radioactive waste

The increasing use of radioisotopes and, more particularly, the development of the nuclear power industry results in an ever-growing quantity of radioactive waste. Continued dispersal of low levels of radioactive waste to the environment means that members of the general population receive radiation exposure from this source. For this reason very strict control is exercised over the release of radioactive waste to the environment, see Chapter 11. At present the contribution to the total exposure of members of the population from waste disposal is very low, about 1 μSv/year.

5.8.5 Atmospheric fall-out

In the two decades after the Second World War, several countries undertook atmospheric testing of nuclear weapons. Much of the radioactivity generated by the detonations was injected into the stratosphere (at altitudes of 10–20 km) and distributed around the world by the atmospheric circulation, gradually falling out of the atmosphere onto the surface of the earth over a period of some years. This gives rise to radiation exposure of the population, mainly through contamination of foodstuffs. The nuclides of concern in radioactive fall-out from nuclear weapons testing are similar to those arising from the operation of nuclear power stations. The two most important radionuclides are strontium-90 (^{90}Sr, half-life 28.8 years) and caesium-137 (^{137}Cs, half-life 30.0 years). Strontium-90 concentrates in the skeleton and caesium-137 is distributed uniformly throughout the body.

Although atmospheric testing largely ceased in the 1960s, traces of these radionuclides are still measurable 40 years later because of their relatively long half-lives.

Another source of atmospheric fall-out is radioactivity released into the environment as a result of nuclear accidents, much the largest of which occurred at Chernobyl in the Ukraine in 1986. This, and other accidents are discussed further in Chapter 16.

5.8.6 Occupational exposure

The dose from all occupational exposure, mainly in medicine, industry and research, is very small when averaged over the whole population. The estimated contribution to average dose in the UK is about 6 μSv/year, of which atomic energy workers contribute about 40 per cent with the remainder resulting mainly from medical exposures.

5.9 SUMMARY OF CURRENT SOURCES OF RADIATION

Table 5.2 lists the average annual doses received by members of the public in the UK from the current sources of man-made radiation.

Table 5.2 Average annual doses from man-made radiation in the UK

Source	Dose (mSv/year)
Diagnostic radiology	0.38
Therapeutic radiology	0.03
Radioactive waste	0.001
Fall-out from nuclear weapons	0.006
Occupationally exposed persons	0.006
Other sources	0.005
Approximate total	0.42

SUMMARY OF CHAPTER

Sources of background radiation:

Cosmic radiation originating from the sun and interstellar space. The atmosphere provides shielding.
Radiation from uranium and thorium with their daughter products in the Earth's crust.
Naturally occurring radioactive material (NORM). Material containing enhanced levels of natural radioactivity and which may need protection measures.
Radioactivity in the body. Mainly uranium and thorium plus daughters, and potassium-40.

Man-made sources of radiation:

Medical uses of radiation and radioisotopes for diagnostic and therapeutic purposes. Radioactivity in the environment resulting from discharges of radioactive waste, fall-out from weapons testing and nuclear accidents.
Occupational exposure from nuclear reactors and industrial applications.

REVISION QUESTIONS

1. List the main sources of natural background radiation and discuss how these sources vary with:
   (a) altitude,
   (b) geographical location.
2. Discuss the origins of radon in air and describe how its effects may be ameliorated.
3. Calculate the average dose received by members of the general population (from background radiation) in the UK over the first 30 years of their life.
4. Explain the difference between diagnostic and therapeutic radiology and comment on the contribution of each to the average dose received by members of the public.

The system of radiological protection

6

6.1 THE ROLE OF THE ICRP

The International Commission on Radiological Protection (ICRP) was established by the Second International Congress of Radiology (ICR) in 1928. Since its inception, the ICRP has been the one internationally recognized body responsible for recommending safety standards for radiation protection. It must be emphasized that the ICRP recommendations do not have any direct force of law. However, in most countries of the world the national legislation relating to exposure to radiation is based on the recommendations of the ICRP.

The early recommendations of ICRP were concerned with protection against X-rays and radium. Some of the earliest recommendations dealt with the length of time that a worker should be engaged on radiation work. These were:

1. Not more than 7 h/day.
2. Not more than 5 days/week.
3. Not less than 1 month's holiday per year.
4. Off days to be spent as much as possible out of doors.

The maximum permissible doses were defined very loosely.

In 1950, the ICRP extended its scope to deal with the many new problems resulting from the discovery and exploitation of nuclear fission and the birth of the nuclear industry. Since that time there have been further revisions of the principles of radiological protection and of the dose limits recommended by ICRP. The history of the development of the dose limits for workers is shown in Table 6.1.

All of these changes have led to a decrease in the occupational exposure limits. This continuous decrease has not resulted from any positive evidence of damage to workers exposed within the earlier permissible dose levels, but rather from an increasing awareness of the uncertainties in much of the available experimental data and hence of the need for caution in setting limits.

In early ICRP recommendations the expression **tolerance dose** was used to describe the acceptable level of exposure to radiation. The term tolerance dose had the unfortunate connotation that it seemed to imply a threshold dose below which no radiation damage would occur. On the basis of a growing body of evidence that questioned the existence of a threshold dose for certain types of somatic damage, the term tolerance dose was later

Table 6.1 History of dose limits for workers

Dose limit	Date recommended	Comments
0.1 of an erythema dose per year	1925	Proposed by A. Mutscheller and R. M. Sievert. This corresponds to an exposure of *c.* 30 R/year from 100 kV X-rays or *c.* 70 R/year from 200 kV X-rays
0.2 R/day or 1 R per working week	1934	Recommended by ICRP
150 mSv/year, or approximately 3 mSv/week	1950	Recommended by ICRP
50 mSv/year, or approximately 1 mSv/week	1956	Recommended by ICRP
All exposures to be kept as low as reasonably achievable; equivalent dose limit 50 mSv/year	1977	Recommended by ICRP
Limit of 20 mSv/year on effective dose	1991	Averaging over 5 years permitted subject to the requirement that the dose does not exceed 50 mSv in any one year

ICRP, International Commission on Radiological Protection.

replaced by the term **maximum permissible dose**, which subsequently became simply **dose limit**. However, the important development was that the emphasis changed from working to a dose limit to ensuring that all exposures are kept as low as reasonably achievable within a dose limit. In 1991, the ICRP issued *Publication 60*, containing new basic recommendations within an overall 'System of radiological protection'.

While earlier recommendations were adequate for normal operational conditions, the new system of radiological protection recognized that guidance was needed on two other types of situations:

1. those in which there is the potential but not the certainty of exposure, such as in the case of accidents, or in the disposal of radioactive waste; and
2. those where the source and exposure is pre-existing, or is not under control.

The 1991 recommendations also took account of the most recent epidemiological evidence, particularly the re-evaluation of Japanese data.

In 2003 the ICRP began an extensive period of consultation, aimed at generating a new set of recommendations to replace the 1991 version. Any changes arising from the new recommendations will take some years to be implemented in national legislation and regulations.

6.2 THE 1991 RECOMMENDATIONS OF THE ICRP (*PUBLICATION 60*)

In ICRP *Publication 60*, **practices** are defined as those activities that **add** to the overall radiation exposure, and **interventions** are those that **subtract** from exposure.

For **practices**, the system of protection is based on the following general principles:

1. No practice involving exposure to ionizing radiation should be adopted unless it produces sufficient benefit to the exposed individuals or to society to offset the radiation detriment it causes (**justification of the practice**).
2. In relation to any particular source within a practice, the magnitude of individual doses, the number of people exposed and the likelihood of incurring exposures that are not certain to be received shall be kept as low as reasonably achievable, economic and social factors being taken into account. This procedure should be subject to dose or risk **constraints** to limit the inequity likely to result from economic and social judgements (**optimization of protection**).
3. The exposure of individuals resulting from the combination of all relevant practices should be subject to dose or risk limits (**dose and risk limitation**).

The concept of constraints to dose or risk is intended to ensure that limits are not exceeded as a result of exposure to several sources. The constraints relate to individuals but are applied to a single source. For example, if members of a population could receive exposure from several different sources, constraints would need to be applied to each source so as to ensure that the total exposure of any individual remained within the overall dose limit.

For **intervention**, the system of protection is based on the following general principles:

1. Any intervention must do more good than harm.
2. The scale and duration of the intervention should be such that the net benefit should be as large as reasonably achievable.

As an example of intervention, consider the case of a site that has been contaminated by previous industrial operations, possibly many decades ago when no standards were applied to the release of the site, and has subsequently been used for other purposes. A decision to clean up the site would represent an intervention and the purpose would be to reduce the levels of exposure of those using the site in the future. In making the decision to clean up the site, it would need to be established that the exposure arising from the clean up (including the disposal of the radioactive material from the site) would not exceed that which would occur in the future if the site was not cleaned up.

A summary and review of information on the biological effects of ionizing radiation are included in ICRP *Publication 60* and, on the basis of the review, quantitative estimates are made of the consequences of radiation exposure, as discussed in Chapter 4. Estimates are made for both **stochastic** and **deterministic** effects. To reiterate:

Stochastic effects are those for which the probability of an effect occurring, rather than its severity, is regarded as a function of dose, without threshold. The most important somatic stochastic effect is the induction of cancers, for which the risk must be regarded as increasing progressively with increasing dose received, without threshold. Similarly, at the dose levels involved in radiation protection, genetic effects are regarded as being stochastic.

Deterministic effects are those for which the severity of the effect varies with the dose, and for which a threshold may exist. Examples of deterministic injuries are cataract of the lens of the eye, damage to blood vessels and impairment of fertility. The severity of these effects varies with the size of the radiation dose received but they are not detectable at all unless a quite high threshold dose is exceeded.

The aim of radiation protection, as stated by the ICRP, is to prevent detrimental deterministic effects and to limit the probability of stochastic effects to levels deemed to be acceptable. This aim is achieved by:

1. Setting dose limits at levels that are sufficiently low to ensure that no threshold dose is reached, even following exposure for the whole of an individual's lifetime – **prevention of deterministic effects**.
2. Keeping all justifiable exposures as low as is reasonably achievable, economic and social factors being taken into account, subject always to the boundary condition that the appropriate dose limits shall not be exceeded – **limitation of stochastic effects**.

In *Publication 60*, the ICRP considered three levels related to the degree of tolerability of an exposure or risk. These are unacceptable, tolerable and acceptable. A limit represents a selected boundary in the region between 'unacceptable' and 'tolerable' levels. Tolerable implies that the exposure (or risk) is not welcomed, but can reasonably be tolerated, and acceptable means that the level of protection has been optimized and can be accepted without further improvement. The dose limits therefore represent the level at which continued exposure would be only just tolerable.

6.3 RECOMMENDED DOSE LIMITS FOR WORKERS

To limit stochastic effects the ICRP recommends an annual effective dose limit for uniform irradiation of the whole body of 20 mSv, averaged over a period of 5 years. It is permissible to exceed 20 mSv in any one year but the dose should not exceed 50 mSv in any year. For non-uniform irradiation of the body, weighting factors have been assigned to the various individual organs, relative to the whole body as 1.0, reflecting the harm attributable to irradiation of each organ. The sum of the weighted organ doses is known as the **effective dose**, E. Thus:

$$E = \sum_T w_T H_T$$

where w_T is the weighting factor for tissue T and H_T is the equivalent dose in tissue T. The annual limit on effective dose is 20 mSv and so in any one year

$$\sum_T w_T H_T \leq 20\,\text{mSv}$$

The weighting factors are given in Table 6.2.

The use of an annual effective dose limit of 20 mSv implies that, if the conditions of exposure were such that only a single tissue T were exposed, the limiting annual equivalent dose for that tissue would be:

$$\text{Dose limit}_T = 20/w_T\,\text{mSv}$$

For example, in the case of the lung, w_T has a value of 0.12, and this implies an annual limit on equivalent dose to the lung of about 170 mSv. Similarly, for the thyroid w_T has a

Table 6.2 Tissue weighting factors

Tissue or organ	Tissue weighting factor, w_T
Gonads	0.20
Bone marrow (red)	0.12
Colon	0.12
Lung	0.12
Stomach	0.12
Bladder	0.05
Breast	0.05
Liver	0.05
Oesophagus	0.05
Thyroid	0.05
Skin	0.01
Bone surface	0.01
Remainder	0.05

The values are averages across a population of all ages and both sexes. They may be applied to workers and to members of the public.

EXAMPLE 6.1

Calculate the allowable equivalent dose to the thyroid of a worker for a year in which he is exposed to non-uniform irradiation involving the whole body and the lung, as well as the thyroid. During the year he receives equivalent doses of 10 mSv to the whole body and 50 mSv to the lung.
  Using the weighting factor formula:

$$\sum_T w_T H_T \leq 20 \text{ mSv}$$

w_T (whole body) $\times$ H_T (whole body) + w_T (lung) $\times$ H_T (lung) + w_T (thyroid) $\times$ H_T (thyroid) $\leqslant$ 20 mSv.

Thus,

  1.0×10 mSv $+ 0.12 \times 50$ mSv $+ 0.05 \times H_T$ (thyroid) $= 20$ mSv, in the limit

i.e.

  10 mSv $+$ 6 mSv $+$ 0.05 H_T (thyroid) $= 20$ mSv

  H_T (thyroid) $= \frac{20 - 16}{0.05} = 80$ mSv

Thus the worker is permitted to receive up to 80 mSv equivalent dose to the thyroid during the year in question.

---

value of 0.05 and so the annual equivalent dose limit for the thyroid is 400 mSv. For most of the organs and tissues of the body the 'stochastic' equivalent dose limits are lower than the threshold doses at which deterministic effects start to occur (generally about 500 mSv although a few tissues show higher radiosensitivities). Thus the restrictions on effective dose are sufficient to ensure the avoidance of deterministic effects in almost all tissues and organs. The exceptions are the skin and the hands and the feet, for which an equivalent dose limit of 500 mSv in one year is recommended, and the lens of the eye, for which a limit of 150 mSv/year is recommended.

EXAMPLE 6.2

Using the weighting factors in Table 6.2, calculate the implied limits for the gonads and the thyroid, assuming that each organ is irradiated completely in isolation.

For gonads, $w_T = 0.20$, and so

implied annual limit $= \frac{20}{0.2} = 100$ mSv

For thyroid, $w_T = 0.05$, thus

implied annual limit $= \frac{20}{0.05} = 400$ mSv

6.4 NOTES ON THE DOSE LIMITS FOR WORKERS

The following points should be stressed in applying this system of dose limitation:

1. All unnecessary exposures should be avoided.
2. While it is permissible to average a worker's dose over 5 years, the effective dose should not exceed 50 mSv in any single year.
3. The Commission lays considerable emphasis on the fact that only a few workers would be expected to receive annual doses close to the recommended limit. Experience shows that in many industries the distribution of doses has often been such that the average worker has received an annual whole-body equivalent dose of about 2 mSv. Using the risk factors quoted in *Publication 60* this implies that the average risk of death in such occupations involving radiation exposure is comparable with the average risk in other industries which are normally considered 'safe'.
4. The basis for control of the occupational exposure of women is the same as for men except that when a pregnancy is declared, a supplementary equivalent dose limit of 2 mSv to the surface of the abdomen should apply to the remainder of the pregnancy.
5. Work places should be subject to classification:
   Controlled area – in which normal working conditions require workers to follow well-established procedures.
   Supervised area – where no special procedures are normally needed but practices are kept under review.

6.5 RECOMMENDED DOSE LIMITS FOR INDIVIDUAL MEMBERS OF THE PUBLIC

In *Publication 60*, the ICRP recommends an annual effective dose limit of 1 mSv for individual members of the public. However, they also recommend that, in special circumstances, a higher value of effective dose could be allowed in a single year, provided that the average over 5 years does not exceed 1 mSv/year. To prevent deterministic effects, the ICRP recommends dose limits of 15 mSv/year for the lens of the eye and 50 mSv/year for the skin (Table 6.3).

Table 6.3 Recommended dose limits*

	Dose limit	
	Occupational	Public
Effective dose	20 mSv per year, averaged over defined period of 5 years[†]	1 mSv in a year[‡]
Annual equivalent dose in:[§]		
lens of the eye	150 mSv	15 mSv
skin	500 mSv	50 mSv
hands and feet	500 mSv	–

*The limits apply to the sum of the relevant doses from external exposure in the specified period and the 50-year committed dose (to age 70 years for children) from intakes in the same period. [†]The effective dose should not exceed 50 mSv in any single year. [‡]In special circumstances, a higher value of effective dose could be allowed in a single year, provided that the average over 5 years does not exceed 1 mSv per year. [§]For other organs, stochastic effects are limiting and hence the dose to these other organs is controlled by the limit on effective dose.

6.6 ABNORMAL EXPOSURES IN EMERGENCIES OR ACCIDENTS

In an emergency, volunteers may receive large doses for the purpose of saving life or preventing serious injuries, or to prevent a substantial increase in the scale of the incident. It is difficult to specify limits to cover such an event since each situation will be unique. When rescue operations have to be undertaken, it may not be possible to work to specified dose limits. Each situation must be assessed by those responsible for the operations, and a decision reached on the basis of this assessment.

To limit the exposure of workers and the general public following an accidental release of radioactive material it is necessary to have a detailed and well-rehearsed emergency plan. The emergency plan has three objectives:

1. To restrict exposures as far as is reasonably achievable and, in particular, to attempt to avoid exposures above the dose limits.
2. To bring the situation back under control.
3. To obtain information for assessing the causes and consequences of the incident.

The ICRP considers that occupational exposures of emergency teams during remedial actions can be limited by operational controls. In the case of serious accidents the controls could be relaxed but this should not result in exposures of more than about 0.5 Sv (or 5 Sv to skin), except for life-saving actions.

It is usually considered that whole-body doses of up to about 1 Sv could be justifiable in the saving of life. If the operation would require doses much in excess of this level, then the risks and possible result of the operation would have to be judged very carefully. One important consideration would be the accuracy of the information regarding the likely dose rates in the accident area; a second would be the condition of the casualties and their likelihood of survival.

Regarding exposure of members of the public following an accident, the ICRP believes that it is not possible for them to fix generally applicable intervention levels above which intervention by the appropriate authorities would always be required. All countermeasures that can be applied to reduce the exposure of members of the public following an accidental release of radioactive materials, such as sheltering, taking stable iodine tablets or evacuation, carry some detriment to the people concerned. Thus the decision to introduce countermeasures (i.e. make an intervention) must be based on a balance of the detriment which they carry and the reduction in the exposure that they are likely to achieve.

However, the ICRP judges that it might be possible to set levels below which intervention would not generally be considered to be justified. Such intervention levels and derived intervention levels should be included in an emergency plan, which should also give guidance on the different countermeasures available. It is emphasized that the emergency plan should be sufficiently flexible to allow its adaptation to the real accident situation. In particular, the intervention levels should not be applied in an automatic fashion but should be reassessed in the light of the available information at the time of intervention.

SUMMARY OF CHAPTER

International Commission on Radiological Protection (ICRP): internationally recognized body responsible for recommending a system of radiological protection.

Stochastic effects: those for which the probability of an effect occurring, rather than its severity, is regarded as a function of dose, without threshold (e.g. cancer induction or genetic effects).

Deterministic effects: those for which the severity of the effect varies with the dose, and for which a threshold may therefore apply (e.g. cataracts of the lens of the eye, damage to blood vessels or impairment of fertility).

Aim of ICRP recommendations: to prevent detrimental deterministic effects and to limit the probability of stochastic effects to acceptable levels.

Deterministic dose limit: 0.5 Sv in 1 year for the skin and for hands and feet, 0.15 Sv for the lens of the eye.

Stochastic dose limit: an effective dose of 20 mSv/year averaged over a defined period of 5 years, with no more than 50 mSv in any one year; for non-uniform irradiation, apply the formula

$$\sum_{T} w_T H_T \leq 20\,\text{mSv}$$

with the appropriate weighting factors (w_T) for individual organs.

Controlled area: in which workers are required to follow well-established procedures.

Supervised area: in which special procedures are not normally needed but where the situation is kept under review.

Dose limits for individual members of the public: lifetime annual average effective dose limit is 1 mSv. Subsidiary annual dose limit of 5 mSv for some years, subject to lifetime average not being exceeded.

Emergency exposures:

1. Attempt to avoid exposures above the dose limits.
2. In serious accidents, controls may be relaxed but should not result in exposures of more than about 0.5 Sv (or 5 Sv to skin).

3. It may be justifiable to allow doses up to about 1 Sv for saving a life.
4. Intervention levels to reduce exposures of public.

REVISION QUESTIONS

1. Explain the main features of the system of radiological protection recommended by the ICRP in its *Publication 60*.
2. Explain what is meant by the terms stochastic and deterministic effects and give two examples of each type of effect.
3. Give the annual deterministic limit (for workers) for each of the following: the lens of the eye; the hands; the feet.
4. Explain how the doses to various organs of the body from non-uniform irradiation are related to the whole-body limit for uniform irradiation.
5. A worker is required to work in an area where he is subjected to non-uniform irradiation, involving exposure of the whole body, the red bone marrow and the lung. During 1 year the following equivalent doses are received:

whole body	10 mSv
lung	100 mSv
red bone marrow	150 mSv

   Calculate the committed effective dose.
6. Assuming, in turn, that each of the following organs of a worker is irradiated for the entire year in isolation, calculate the annual dose limit implied for each organ by the weighting factor formula: the breast, the red bone marrow, the lung and the thyroid.
7. State the main differences between controlled and supervised areas.
8. Explain the main considerations that should be applied to the exposure of workers and members of the public in an accident or an emergency. Why might it sometimes be permissible, following an accident, for workers to be exposed in excess of the normal operational control limits?

Radiation detection and measurement

7.1 GENERAL PRINCIPLES

The fact that the human body is unable to sense ionizing radiation is probably responsible for much of the general apprehension about this type of hazard. Reliance must be placed on detection devices which are based on the physical or chemical effects of radiation. These effects include:

- ionization in gases;
- ionization and excitation in certain solids;
- changes in chemical systems; and
- activation by neutrons.

The majority of health physics monitoring instruments use detectors based on ionization of a gas. Certain classes of crystalline solids exhibit increases in electrical conductivity and effects attributable to excitation, including scintillation, thermoluminescence and the photographic effect. Detection systems are available in which chemical changes are measured but these are rather insensitive. A method which may be applied to neutron detection depends on the activation caused by neutron reactions.

In this chapter, the basic principles of those systems commonly used in practical health physics are described. Their applications to particular types of measurement are covered in Chapters 8, 9 and 15.

7.2 IONIZATION OF A GAS

7.2.1 Ionization chamber

It will be recalled from Chapter 3 that the absorption of radiation in a gas results in the production of ion pairs consisting of a **negative ion** (the electron) and a **positive ion**. A moderate voltage applied between two plates (electrodes) in close proximity causes the negative ions to be attracted to the positive electrode (anode) and the positive ions to the negative electrode (cathode). This flow of ions constitutes an electric current which is a measure of the intensity of radiation in the gas volume. The current is extremely low (typically about 10^{-12} amperes) and a sensitive electronic circuit known as a direct current amplifier is used to measure it. This system is known as an **ionization chamber** and the current measured is a mean value owing to the interaction of many charged particles or photons (Fig. 7.1).

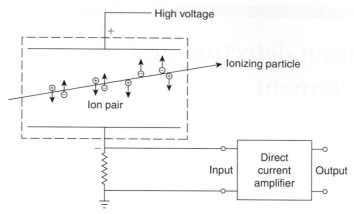

FIGURE 7.1 Ion chamber system.

The design of the chamber and the choice of filling gas depend on the particular application. In health physics instruments the chamber is usually filled with air and is constructed of materials with low atomic number. If the instrument is required to respond to β radiation, which has a very short range in solids, the chamber must have thin walls or a thin entrance window.

7.2.2 Proportional counter

If, in an ion chamber system, the applied voltage is increased beyond a certain point, an effect known as **gas amplification** occurs. This is because the electrons produced by ionization are accelerated by the applied voltage to a sufficiently high energy to cause further ionization themselves before reaching the anode, and a cascade of ionization results (Fig. 7.2). Thus, a single ionizing particle or photon can produce a pulse of current that is large enough to be detected. Over a certain range of voltage the size of the pulse is proportional to the amount of energy deposited by the original particle or photon and so the system is known as a **proportional counter**. The term **counter** means that the output is a series of pulses, which may be counted by an appropriate means, rather than an average current as obtained with a direct current ionization chamber.

7.2.3 Geiger–Müller counter

If the voltage in the ionization system is increased still further the gas amplification is so great that a single ionizing particle produces an avalanche of ionization resulting in a very large pulse of current. The size of the pulse is the same, regardless of the quantity of energy initially deposited by the particle or photon, and is governed more by the external circuit than the counter itself. The Geiger–Müller tube is very widely used in monitoring equipment because it is relatively rugged and can directly operate simple output circuits. Again, this is a counting device but it is also possible to use a Geiger–Müller counter in a circuit which measures the average current flowing through the tube.

In practice both proportional and Geiger–Müller counters are usually constructed in the form of a cylinder which forms the cathode, with a central thin wire which is the anode. The whole is enclosed in a glass or metal tube which is filled with a special gas mixture.

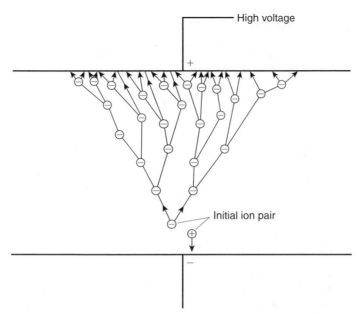

High voltage

+

Initial ion pair

−

FIGURE 7.2 Gas amplification.

7.3 SOLID-STATE DETECTORS

7.3.1 Mechanism

The term **solid-state detectors** refers to certain classes of crystalline substances that exhibit measurable effects when exposed to ionizing radiation. In such substances, electrons exist in definite **energy bands** separated by **forbidden bands**. The highest energy band in which electrons normally exist is the **valence band**. The transfer of energy from a photon or charged particle to a valence electron may raise it from the valence band through the forbidden band into either the **exciton band** or the **conduction band**. The vacancy left by the electron is known as a hole and it is analogous to a positive ion in a gas system.

The raising of an electron to the conduction band is known as ionization and the electron–hole pair can be compared with ion pairs in a gas. The electron and hole are independently mobile and in the presence of an electrical potential will be oppositely attracted, so contributing to electrical conduction in the material. If an electron is raised to the exciton band, the process is excitation. In this case the electron is still bound to the hole by electrical forces and so cannot contribute to conduction. The third process that can occur is **electron trapping**. Traps are imperfections or impurity atoms in the crystal structure which cause electrons to be caught in the forbidden band. The three processes are illustrated in Fig. 7.3.

The existence of the three states may be virtually permanent or they may last a very short time depending on the material and, to a great extent, the temperature. As electrons return to the valence band, the difference in energy is emitted as **fluorescent** radiation, usually a photon of visible light. In the case of trapped electrons, energy must first be provided to enable the electron to escape from the trap back into the exciton band and thence down to the valence band. The energy to release the electrons is usually provided by raising the temperature of the substance; the light given off as a result is known as **thermoluminescence**.

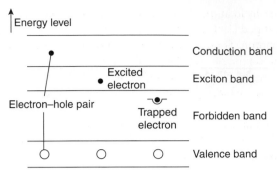

FIGURE 7.3 Ionization, excitation and trapping.

The practical application of the three processes of conductivity, fluorescence and thermo-luminescence is considered in more detail below. It should be mentioned that the photo-graphic effect is also a solid-state process but is treated separately in the following text.

7.3.2 Conductivity detectors

Since changes in conductivity are caused by ionization, solid-state conductivity detectors are similar in some ways to gas ionization systems. A cadmium sulphide (CdS) detector, for example, is analogous to an ion chamber. It is operated in the mean current mode and is suitable in some applications for the measurement of γ dose rate. The main advantage is that it can be much smaller than a gas ionization chamber and yet have a higher sensitivity because of its much greater density.

As with gas systems, some solid-state detectors, notably germanium and silicon, operate in the pulse mode. Germanium has the disadvantage that it must be operated at very low temperatures. The output pulse size in both cases is proportional to the energy deposition of X-rays and γ-rays within the detector. The main application is in gamma spectrometry, in which, by analysing the size of pulses from the detector, it is possible to measure the energy of γ-rays.

7.3.3 Scintillation detectors

Scintillation detectors are based on detection of the fluorescent radiation (usually visible light) emitted when an electron returns from an excited state to the valence band. The material selected is one in which this occurs very quickly (within about 1 μs). The absorption of a 1 MeV γ-photon in a scintillation detector results typically in about 10 000 excitations and a similar number of photons of light. These **scintillations** are detected by means of a photomultiplier tube or photodiode which converts the light into electrical pulses which are then amplified. The size of pulse is proportional to the energy deposited in the crystal by the charged particle or photon. In earlier years, the most common type of scintillator used in γ-ray work was sodium iodide, usually in cylindrical crystals of about 50 mm diameter × 50 mm long. These were widely used in γ-spectrometry and had the advantages of high sensitivity and relatively low cost. They still offer advantages in some applications but have generally been supplanted by germanium detectors which offer better energy resolution. Zinc sulphide crystals in very thin layers are used for α-detection.

7.3.4 Thermoluminescence detectors

Thermoluminescence detectors use the electron trapping process. The material is selected so that electrons trapped as a result of exposure to ionizing radiation are stable at normal temperatures. If, after irradiation, the material is heated to a suitable temperature, usually about 200°C, the trapped electrons are released and return to the valence band with the emission of a light photon. Thus, if the device is heated in the dark under a photomultiplier tube, the light output can be measured and this is proportional to the radiation dose which the detector has received. The most commonly-used material is lithium fluoride but various other materials, including calcium fluoride and lithium borate, are used in special applications.

It should be noted that, while the conductivity and scintillation methods are more suitable for measuring radiation intensity (i.e. dose **rate**), thermoluminescence detectors measure the total dose accumulated over the period of exposure.

7.4 PHOTOGRAPHIC EFFECT

Ionizing radiation affects photographic film in the same way as visible light. A photographic film consists of an emulsion of crystals (grains) of silver bromide on a transparent plastic base. The absorption of energy in a silver bromide grain, whether from light or ionizing radiation, results in the formation of a small cluster (often only a few atoms) of metallic silver. This cluster is known as a **latent image**. When the film is **developed** this tiny amount of silver assists the conversion of all the silver in a grain from its compound form, silver bromide, into metallic silver which deposits on the plastic base material. This is an amplification process with a gain of about 10^9, which accounts for the high sensitivity of photographic emulsions. After development the film is **fixed** or made stable by washing in a sodium thiosulphite (hypo) bath which removes any unconverted silver bromide. If good results are to be obtained it is important to control strictly the developer strength, temperature and processing time.

Photographic films used for radiation monitoring are usually 30×40 mm and are, of course, sealed in a light-tight packet. After processing, the film is read by passing a beam of light through it and measuring the optical density. This observed density is converted to radiation dose by means of a calibration curve obtained by exposing a number of films to known doses and plotting a dose–density curve (see Fig. 7.4).

The sensitivity of the film depends on the grain size of the emulsion. The most sensitive types give a range of dose measurement of about $50\,\mu$Sv to $50\,$mSv.

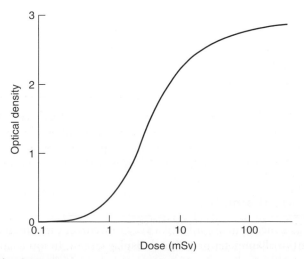

FIGURE 7.4 Dose–density curve.

The main advantage of photographic film is that, with the aid of special film holders incorporating filters, it enables information on the type and energy of radiation to be deduced. In addition, the developed film can be stored and rescrutinized later. The most serious disadvantage is that a rapid reading cannot be obtained.

7.5 ACTIVATION EFFECT

The bombardment of most elements by neutrons produces radioactive nuclides and measurement of the degree of activation permits estimation of the incident neutron flux. In most cases the method is not very sensitive and its main application is in the assessment of large accidental doses.

Fast neutron measurement is often carried out using sulphur discs which undergo the reaction.

$$^{32}S(n, p)^{32}P \quad (P - phosphorus)$$

Other useful reactions for fast neutron measurement include

$$^{115}In(n, \gamma)^{116}In \quad (In - indium)$$

$$^{197}Au(n, \gamma)^{198}Au \quad (Au - gold)$$

The nuclides ^{32}P, ^{116}In and ^{198}Au are β-emitters and are counted in a suitable system.

Another aspect of the activation effect is that a person receiving a large neutron dose (above about 0.1 Gy) would be rendered slightly radioactive and a dose estimate may be made by measurement of the induced activity. For example, activation of sodium (Na) in the body results in the production of ^{24}Na, which is again a β-emitter.

$$^{23}Na(n, \gamma)^{24}Na$$

With moderate doses of neutrons the decay radiation can be detected by simply holding a sensitive detector such as a Geiger–Müller probe against the body.

7.6 ELECTRICAL CIRCUITS

7.6.1 Types of circuit

In Sections 7.2 and 7.3 various detectors were described which give as output an electrical signal. These electrical signals are of two types: direct current and pulse. Measurement of direct current (d.c.) is by d.c. amplifiers, while for pulsed output, counting circuits or ratemeters are used. The important practical features of these circuits are described below.

7.6.2 Direct current amplifier

A d.c. amplifier is a means of amplifying a very low current to a high enough value to operate a conventional ammeter or a digital display circuit. In ion chamber systems the gain required is quite high; the current input may be about 10^{-12} amperes (A) while about

10^{-6} A is necessary to drive a meter. The required gain in this case is 10^6. Amplifiers with such a high gain have a tendency to instability because of temperature fluctuations, etc. This can be reduced to a marked extent by using **negative feedback** (see Fig. 7.5). Briefly, this means that if an increased signal is fed into the input, it results in an opposite signal being fed from the output back to the input. Another important point is that when currents as low as 10^{-12} A are being measured, great care must be taken to prevent stray currents affecting the input. A very high standard of insulation and cleanliness is required between the detector output and the input to the amplifier.

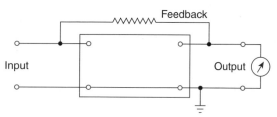

FIGURE 7.5 Direct current amplifier – negative feedback.

The main application of d.c. amplifiers is in ion chamber systems, both portable and fixed, but they are also used for solid-state detectors of the cadmium sulphide type.

7.6.3 Pulse counting systems

A basic counting system consists of a **pulse amplifier**, a **discriminator** and a **scaler**. In addition, the system may contain a **stabilized power supply unit** to provide a supply for the detector.

The function of the pulse amplifier is to accept pulses from the detector and to amplify them to a size compatible with subsequent circuits. The size of pulses depends on the type of detector but is typically a few microvolts for solid-state detectors, a few millivolts for proportional and scintillation counters, and up to a few volts for Geiger–Müller counters. Since most counting circuits operate on pulses of a few volts it will be seen that the amplifier requires a gain of about 10^6 for solid state detectors, 10^3 for proportional and scintillation counters and can operate Geiger–Müller counting circuits directly.

In all electronic apparatus there is present, to some extent, electronic 'noise' in the form of small electrical pulses. These noise pulses are amplified with the signal pulses from the detector and, unless precautions are taken, will be counted by the system. The function of the discriminator is to reject all pulses below a certain level, which is set by applying a **discriminator bias** voltage. The equipment will then record only those pulses whose amplitude exceeds the bias level. Figure 7.6 shows a train of pulses and small noise pulses being fed from an amplifier to a discriminator. If the bias level is reduced below A, noise pulses will be counted and if it is raised above C, detector pulses will not be counted. The correct level is that indicated by B. A discriminator bias characteristic can be plotted by measuring the count rate from a detector with a range of discriminator bias settings. This is illustrated in Fig. 7.7 in which the lines A, B and C correspond to those in the previous figure. Thus if the bias voltage is below A, a very high count rate is recorded and if it exceeds C no counts are recorded. The correct setting is at B at which only genuine pulses from the

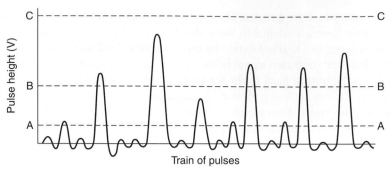

FIGURE 7.6 Function of a discriminator.

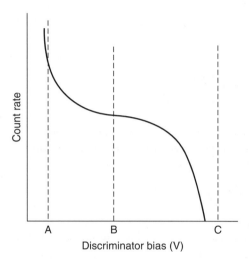

FIGURE 7.7 Discriminator bias characteristic.

detector will be recorded. In addition, since the curve is almost level at this point small variations in the bias setting will not seriously affect the count rate.

The scaler accepts pulses from the discriminator and gives a visual display of the number of pulses (counts) received over the counting period. The scaler usually incorporates a timing device so that once started it will count for a preset time ranging from a few seconds up to a few hours.

The counting rate from detectors is dependent on the voltage applied. To set up the equipment, a small source is placed near the detector and a series of counts made for different detector voltages. The graph obtained by plotting these results is called a plateau because the count rate is relatively independent of the applied voltage over a certain range (see Fig. 7.8). The counter is operated at a voltage between the dotted lines (i.e. on the plateau), so that small variations in supply voltage will not affect the response of the instrument.

A generalized counting system is illustrated in schematic form in Fig. 7.9. The main function of this type of equipment is the measurement of radioactive samples of various types. In health physics the samples evaluated in this way include air sample filter papers, smear and water samples. The practical aspects of sample counting are described in more detail in Chapter 9 and a number of special techniques are given in Chapter 15.

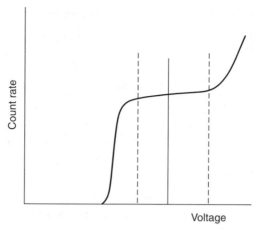

FIGURE 7.8 Plateau for Geiger–Müller counter.

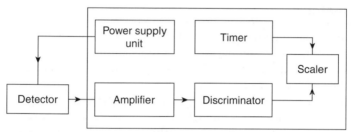

FIGURE 7.9 Counting equipment – schematic diagram.

7.6.4 Pulse height analyser (PHA)

When using detectors from which the output pulse height depends on the energy of the ion-izing particle or photon, it is often of great help to analyse the pulses to obtain information about the radiation spectrum. A pulse height analyser (PHA) separates the pulses into a large number of channels depending on the pulse height. Thus, if the maximum pulse height in a system is 10 V and 100 channels are available, the pulses can be segregated into channels 0.1 V wide. Any pulse smaller than 0.1 V would go into channel 1, pulses of 0.1–0.2 V into channel 2, and so on up to pulses of 9.9–10 V, which would go into channel 100. The num-ber of pulses going into each channel is recorded and presented on a visual display unit in such a way as to give a visual picture of the radiation spectrum. The upper line in Fig. 7.10 shows a cobalt-60 (^{60}Co) γ-ray spectrum as registered by a sodium iodide (NaI) crystal.

The two γ-rays of ^{60}Co really have very precise energies but for various reasons they are 'smeared out' by the NaI detector to give the two rather broad peaks shown. This has the disadvantage that if a sample contains a mixture of radionuclides, the peaks may overlap to some extent, making it difficult to resolve the different energies. Germanium detectors offer advantages in this respect since they give very sharply defined lines and permit pre-cise identification of the γ spectrum and hence the mixture of radionuclides. To take advantage of the high resolution of these detectors, modern PHAs have several thousands of channels.

The lower line in Fig. 7.10 shows the equivalent spectrum obtained from a ^{60}Co source using a germanium detector. A disadvantage of germanium detectors is that they must be maintained at very low temperatures by means of liquid nitrogen cryostats.

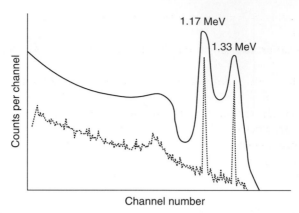

FIGURE 7.10 Cobalt-60 γ-ray spectra from a sodium iodide crystal (solid line) and a germanium (lithium) detector (dotted line).

7.6.5 Ratemeter

If a detector operating in pulse mode is used in portable equipment it is not usually practicable or desirable to use a counting system. A more convenient method of presentation is a ratemeter which accepts pulses and indicates, either on a conventional meter or digital display, a reading related to the pulse rate.

A basic ratemeter circuit is shown in Fig. 7.11. Each pulse feeds a charge into the capacitor C, which then slowly discharges through the resistance R, giving a reading on the meter. The reading on the meter or display constantly fluctuates because the arrival of a new pulse causes a sudden increase in reading followed by a slow decrease until the next pulse arrives. The degree of fluctuation can be reduced by increasing the time constant of the circuit, which means increasing the value of C or R, or both of them. The time constant in seconds is obtained by multiplying C (farads) by R (ohms). Although an increase of time constant smoothes out the meter reading it also slows down the response of the circuit to sudden changes in pulse rate. After a change in pulse rate it takes about four time constants for the ratemeter to show the new reading. For portable monitoring equipment the time constant should not normally exceed 3 s or so.

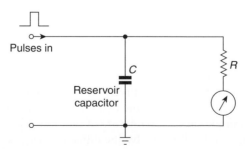

FIGURE 7.11 Basic ratemeter circuit.

SUMMARY OF CHAPTER

Ionization in gases: measured by ion chamber system with current output.
Gas amplification: ionization electrons cause further ionization if the voltage applied is high enough.

Proportional counter: gives pulses of current proportional to amount of energy deposited by original particle.

Geiger–Müller counter: each single ionizing particle causes an avalanche of electrons that gives a pulse output.

Solid-state detectors: rely on ionization, excitation and electron trapping in special crystalline substances.

Conductivity detectors: may be used in pulse or current mode.

Scintillation counters: detect light pulses from scintillator using a photomultiplier tube.

Thermoluminescent detectors: energy stored until material is heated, then light emitted. Provides rapid read-out.

Photographic effect: blackening of film, dose–density curve. Provides permanent dose record.

Activation effect: measures activation caused by neutrons.

Direct current: amplifier measures low currents.

Pulse counting systems: consist of pulse amplifier, discriminator, scaler.

Pulse height analysers: show the radiation spectrum.

Ratemeter: registers pulse rate on a meter or digital display.

REVISION QUESTIONS

1. Describe the operation of a Geiger–Müller counter.
2. Which class of solid-state detector is suitable for measuring a person's accumulated radiation dose? How does the detector function?
3. Write a short description of the photographic effect and discuss its advantages and disadvantages in personal dosimetry.
4. Draw a schematic diagram of a counting system and describe briefly the function of the various circuits.

The external radiation hazard   8

8.1 SOURCE OF THE HAZARD

The **external radiation hazard** arises from sources of radiation outside the body. When radioactive material actually gets inside the body it gives rise to an **internal radiation hazard**, which requires quite different methods of control. The internal radiation hazard is discussed in Chapter 9.

The external hazard may be from β, X, γ or neutron radiation, all of which can penetrate to the sensitive organs of the body. Alpha radiation is not normally regarded as an external radiation hazard as it cannot penetrate the outer layers of the skin. The external hazard is controlled by applying the three principles: **time, distance** and **shielding**.

8.2 TIME

The dose accumulated by a person working in an area having a particular dose rate is directly proportional to the amount of time they spend in the area. The dose can thus be controlled by limiting the time spent in the area, as defined by the equation:

$$\text{Dose} = \text{dose rate} \times \text{time}$$

EXAMPLE 8.1

The annual dose limit for workers is 20 mSv per year which, assuming a 50-week working year, corresponds to 0.4 mSv, or 400 μSv per week. How many hours can a worker spend each week in an area in which the dose rate is 20 μSv/h?

$$\text{Dose} = \text{dose rate} \times \text{time}$$

$$400 = 20 \times t$$

$$\therefore t = 20 \text{ h}$$

EXAMPLE 8.2

If a worker has to spend a full 40-h working week in a particular area, what is the maximum dose rate which can be allowed?

$$\text{Dose} = \text{dose rate} \times \text{time}$$

$$400 = \text{dose rate} \times 40$$

$$\therefore \text{dose rate} = 10 \ \mu\text{Sv/h}$$

EXAMPLE 8.3

What would be the annual dose to a worker who spends a full working year (say 2000 h) in an area where the average dose rate is 2.5 μSv/h?

$$\text{Dose} = \text{dose rate} \times \text{time}$$

$$= 2.5 \times 2000$$

$$= 5000 \ \mu\text{Sv (or 5 mSv)}$$

EXAMPLE 8.4

The dose limit for individual members of the public is 1 mSv/year. What is the maximum dose rate permitted in an area that could be continuously occupied (i.e. 168 h/week) by members of the public? (Answer: ~0.12 μSv/h)

From these Examples 1–4 it can be seen that the dose rates which are of particular interest and which are commonly encountered in and around facilities such as nuclear reactors range from about 0.1 μSv/h up to a few tens of μSv/h. However, it should not be inferred from the examples that the only requirement is that the dose should be less than the dose limit. As discussed in Chapter 6, it is required that, within the limits, doses are as low as reasonably achievable (ALARA). This involves analysing the situation to see if the sources of exposure or the time spent by workers in the area can be reduced. It also requires that means of reducing the dose rate need to be considered. The available methods are: increase the distance between the worker and the source of radiation, or introduce some shielding material between the worker and the radiation source.

8.3 DISTANCE

Consider a point source of radiation which is emitting uniformly in all directions. It was shown in Chapter 3 that the flux at a distance r from a point source is inversely proportional to the square of the distance r. Since the radiation dose rate is directly related to flux it follows that the dose rate also obeys the inverse square law. It should be noted that this is only strictly true for a point source, a point detector and negligible absorption of radiation between source and detector. The inverse square law may be written:

$$D \propto 1/r^2 \quad \text{or} \quad D = k/r^2$$

$$\therefore Dr^2 = k$$

where k is a constant for a particular source

$$\therefore D_1 r_1^2 = D_2 r_2^2$$

where

D_1 = dose rate at distance r_1 from the source
D_2 = dose rate at distance r_2 from the source

EXAMPLE 8.5

The dose rate at 2 m from a particular gamma source is 400 μSv/h. At what distance will it give a dose rate of 25 μSv/h?

$$D_1 r_1^2 = D_2 r_2^2$$

$$400 \times 2^2 = 25 \times r_2^2$$

$$\therefore r_2^2 = 64$$

$$\text{and } r_2 = 8 \text{ m}$$

It will be noted that doubling the distance from the source reduces the dose rate to one-quarter of its original value, trebling the distance reduces the dose rate to one-ninth, and so on.

8.3.1 Expression for calculating the dose rate from γ sources

A useful expression for calculating the approximate dose rate from a γ source is:

$$D = \frac{ME}{6r^2}$$

where

D = dose rate in μSv/h
M = activity of the source in MBq
E = γ energy per disintegration in MeV
r = distance from the source in metres

When applying this expression, care is needed in selecting the correct units. It must be emphasized that in any real situation, protection should be based on measurements of the dose rate.

EXAMPLE 8.6

Calculate the approximate dose rate at a distance of 2 m from a 240-MBq cobalt-60 source. Cobalt-60 emits two γ-rays per disintegration, of 1.17 MeV and 1.33 MeV.

$$D = \frac{ME}{6r^2} \,\mu\text{Sv/h}$$

$$= \frac{240 \times (1.17 + 1.33)}{6 \times 2^2}$$

$$= \frac{240 \times 2.5}{24}$$

$$= 25 \,\mu\text{Sv/h}$$

EXAMPLE 8.7

Calculate the activity of a sodium-22 (^{22}Na) source which gives a dose rate of 64 μSv/h at 1 m. ^{22}Na emits one γ-photon of energy 1.28 MeV per disintegration. (Answer: 300 MBq)

8.4 SHIELDING

The third method of controlling the external radiation hazard is by means of shielding. Generally, this is the preferred method because it results in intrinsically safe working conditions, while reliance on distance or time of exposure may involve continuous administrative control over workers.

The amount of shielding required depends on the type of radiation, the activity of the source and on the dose rate which is acceptable outside the shielding material.

Alpha particles are very easily absorbed. A thin sheet of paper is usually sufficient to stop α particles and so they never present a shielding problem.

Beta radiation is more penetrating than α radiation. In the energy range which is normally encountered (up to about 4 MeV) β radiation requires shielding of up to 10 mm of Perspex for complete absorption. The ease with which β sources may be shielded sometimes leads to the erroneous impression that they are not as dangerous as γ or neutron sources and that large open β sources may be handled directly. This is an extremely dangerous practice as, for instance, the absorbed dose rate at a distance of 3 mm from a β source of 1 MBq is about 1 Gy/h.

A significant problem, encountered when shielding against β radiation, is the emission of secondary X-rays, which result from the rapid slowing down of the β particles and which are more penetrating than the β radiation. This X radiation is known as **bremsstrahlung** and will be discussed more fully in Chapter 12. The fraction of β energy reappearing as bremsstrahlung is approximately $ZE/3000$ where Z is the atomic number of the absorber and E is the β-energy in MeV. This means that β shields should be constructed of materials of low mass number (e.g. aluminium or Perspex) to reduce the amount of bremsstrahlung emitted.

A β source emits β particles with energies covering the complete spectrum from zero up to a characteristic maximum energy, E_{max}. The mean β energy is, in most cases, about $\frac{1}{3}E_{max}$. The penetrating power of β particles depends on their energy. This fact can be used to estimate the energy of the β radiation to aid identification of an unknown source. This will be discussed in more detail in Chapter 15.

Gamma and X radiations are attenuated exponentially when they pass through any material. The dose rate resulting from X- or γ radiation emerging from a shield can be written as:

$$D_t = D_0 e^{-\mu t}$$

where

D_0 = dose rate without shielding
D_t = dose rate after passing through a shield of thickness t
μ = linear absorption coefficient of the material of the shield.

The linear absorption coefficient μ is a function of the type of material used for the shield and also of the energy of the incident photons. It has the dimensions of $(length)^{-1}$ and is usually expressed in m^{-1} or mm^{-1}.

8.4.1 Half-value layer

The half thickness or half-value layer (HVL) for a particular shielding material is the thickness required to reduce the intensity to one half its incident value. Writing the half-value layer as $t_{\frac{1}{2}}$, the previous equation becomes:

$$\frac{D_t}{D_0} = 0.5 = \exp(-\mu t_{\frac{1}{2}})$$

Taking logs to the base e:

$$\log_e 0.5 = -\mu t_{\frac{1}{2}}$$
$$\therefore -0.693 = -\mu t_{\frac{1}{2}}$$
$$\therefore t_{\frac{1}{2}} = \frac{0.693}{\mu}$$

The concept of HVL is very useful in doing rapid, approximate shielding calculations. One HVL reduces the intensity to one-half, two HVLs reduce the intensity to one-quarter, three HVLs to one-eighth and so on, as illustrated in Fig. 8.1.

The value of μ, and hence $t_{\frac{1}{2}}$, depends on the material of the medium and on the radiation energy.

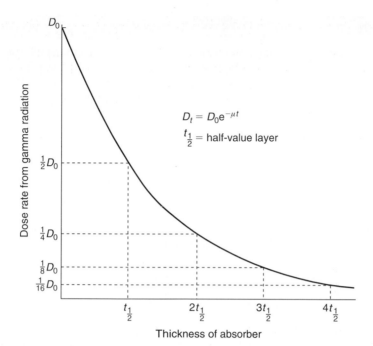

FIGURE 8.1 Variation of γ dose rate with absorber thickness.

Another value sometimes used in shielding work is the **tenth-value layer**, $t_{1/10}$. By a calculation similar to that carried out above it can be shown that:

$$t_{1/10} = \frac{\log_e(10)}{\mu} = \frac{2.303}{\mu}$$

Some typical values of $t_{1/2}$ and $t_{1/10}$ for lead and water are given in Table 8.1.

Table 8.1 Approximate values of $t_{1/2}$ and $t_{1/10}$

γ Radiation energy(MeV)	Millimetres of lead		Millimetres of water	
	$t_{1/2}$	$t_{1/10}$	$t_{1/2}$	$t_{1/10}$
0.5	4	12.5	150	500
1.0	11	35	190	625
1.5	15	50	210	700
2.0	19	60	225	750

EXAMPLE 8.8

The dose rate close to a valve is 160 μSv/h. If this is caused by cobalt-60 inside the valve, how much lead shielding must be placed around the valve to reduce the dose rate to 10 μSv/h? The HVL of lead for ^{60}Co γ radiation is 12.5 mm.

It is required to reduce the dose rate from 160 μSv/h to 10 μSv/h, i.e. by a factor of 16. To do this will require four HVL of lead ($2 \times 2 \times 2 \times 2 = 16$), therefore 4×12.5 mm of lead are required, i.e. 50 mm.

EXAMPLE 8.9

A certain cobalt-60 source gives a dose rate of 40 μSv/h at 1 m. At what distance from the source must a barrier be placed if the dose rate at the barrier must not exceed 2.5 μSv/h? What thickness of lead would give the same protection at the original distance? (HVL of lead for ^{60}Co γ radiation is 12.5 mm.)
   (Answer: 4 m; 50 mm of lead)

Neutron shielding is complicated by the very wide range of neutron energies generally encountered. This means that any shielding equipment has to take account of a number of different, energy-related reactions, the most important of which are:

1. **Elastic scatter**, in which the neutron collides with the target nucleus and 'bounces' off it in a manner similar to the collision of two billiard balls. During the collision, the neutron loses some of its initial energy and this energy is transferred to the target nucleus. All of this transferred energy appears as kinetic energy of the target nucleus. Light elements are best for slowing down neutrons by elastic scatter and so materials with a high hydrogen content (such as paraffin, water, concrete) are used.
2. **Inelastic scatter**; in this process the incoming neutrons impart some of their energy to the scattering material and excite the target nuclei. These target nuclei usually emit γ radiation later when they return to their ground state. The inelastic scatter process is most important for heavy nuclei.
3. **Neutron capture** reactions of many kinds; in these reactions neutrons are captured by nuclei which then de-excite by emitting another particle or photon. One very important neutron capture reaction is:

$$^{10}B(n, \alpha)^7Li$$

The importance of this reaction, from a shielding point of view, lies in the fact that the emitted α particle is very easily absorbed. Thus, the incorporation of boron-10 in shields means that neutrons are absorbed and the resulting α particles cause no further shielding problems.

Unfortunately, the most common neutron-capture reactions lead to the emission of penetrating γ radiation, for example

$$^{58}Fe(n, \gamma)^{59}Fe$$

Capture γ radiation is usually a limitation in shield design and a material of high atomic number is often incorporated to absorb capture γ radiation.

The neutron reactions are illustrated schematically in Fig. 8.2.

8.5 NEUTRON SOURCES

Nuclear fission reactors are the source of large fluxes of neutrons(see Chapter 10). However, there are simpler methods for producing relatively small neutron sources. The most commonly-used depend on the reaction:

$$^9Be(\alpha, n)^{12}C$$

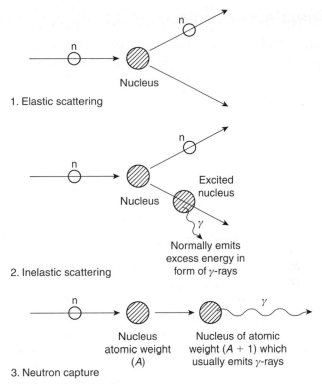

FIGURE 8.2 The three main neutron reactions.

A typical neutron source of this type consists of a quantity of the element beryllium mixed with an α-emitting radionuclide, usually americium-241 (^{241}Am), in a sealed capsule. For ^{241}Am–^{9}Be sources, the source strength is about 70 neutrons per second per MBq of ^{241}Am. The spectrum of neutrons emitted from an α-beryllium source is not monoenergetic but is highly peaked at energies between 3 MeV and 6 MeV; in other words, these neutron sources produce mainly fast neutrons.

Another reaction used to produce neutrons is the photoneutron process, that is the (γ, n) reaction. The most common type of photoneutron source consists of a mixture of equal volumes of antimony and beryllium, in which high energy γ-rays from antimony-124 interact with beryllium nuclei causing the ejection of neutrons. It is worth noting that the neutrons produced by the (γ, n) process are, for most practical purposes, monoenergetic.

To calculate the flux at a distance r from a source of strength Q, the following expression is used (see Chapter 3):

$$\Phi = \frac{Q}{4\pi r^2}$$

EXAMPLE 8.10

Calculate the dose equivalent rate at 1 m from a 0.1 TBq americium–beryllium source (1 TBq of ^{241}Am–Be emits 7×10^7 n/s). Assume that 10^4 n/(m²s) is equivalent to 1 µSv/h. (Answer: 56 µSv/h)

8.6 PERSONAL DOSE CONTROL

Routine control of personal dose is based on a system of area classification. Various systems and terminologies are in use. The basic objective is to segregate areas according to the radiological hazard. In areas where the exposure is unlikely to exceed one-tenth of the dose limit for exposed workers, i.e. 2 mSv/year, no special arrangements are necessary. Where workers could exceed this level of exposure, but are unlikely to exceed three-tenths of the dose limit, i.e. 6 mSv/year, the area would be classified as a **supervised area**. Areas in which exposure could exceed three-tenths of the dose limit are called **controlled areas**. Workers who routinely have access to controlled areas, or who are liable to exceed 6 mSv/year are known as category A workers. All other exposed workers are known as category B workers. Within controlled areas there may be regions where further demarcation is required to avoid over-exposure. In some establishments these are called **restricted areas**.

A typical system of classification considers four types of area:

1. **Uncontrolled areas**, in which the dose rate does not exceed 1 μSv/h. Personnel can work for 40 h/week and 50 weeks/year without exceeding 2 mSv/year.
2. **Supervised areas**, in which the dose rate does not generally exceed 3 μSv/h and hence, in which personnel will not exceed three-tenths of the dose limit. As implied by the name, these areas are subject to some form of supervision, and personnel working regularly in such areas could be subject to routine personal monitoring.
3. **Controlled areas**, in which the dose rate exceeds 3 μSv/h. Personnel working regularly in controlled areas are designated as category A workers and are subject to medical supervision and routine personal monitoring.
4. **Restricted areas**, in which the dose rate exceeds 10 μSv/h. Access to these areas would be subject to special precautions, such as limitation of access time and the use of protective equipment and monitoring devices.

When operating a system of area classification it is necessary to survey the area regularly to confirm that the classification of the area is correct and that adequate precautions are being taken. In controlled and restricted areas, personal dosemeters such as film badges or thermoluminescent dosemeters (TLD) must be worn to measure the accumulated dose to the worker. In addition, a direct reading dosemeter such as an electronic personal dosemeter is often worn to give on-the-spot control.

8.7 RADIATION SURVEY MONITORING

8.7.1 Radiation survey monitoring

This is carried out:

1. During commissioning of a facility to test the adequacy of the shielding and to show that the radiation levels are satisfactory.
2. Whenever changes are made which could affect radiation levels, such as changes in layout or shielding arrangements.
3. Routinely, during operation, to determine the working radiation levels to control accumulated dose.

The ideal radiation survey monitor should be capable of monitoring all forms of penetrating radiation, it should be portable, easy to use and indicate effective dose rate. In practice it is not possible to design a single instrument to fulfil all these requirements and so different instruments have been developed for different types of radiation.

8.7.2 X and γ radiation monitors

One type of radiation monitor measures X and γ radiation and sometimes has a facility to permit an indication (usually not very accurate) of β radiation. The actual method of detection depends on the sensitivity required. Ion chambers can only be used down to levels of a few tens of μSv/h; below this level the size of chamber required is too large for portable instruments. Increased sensitivity is obtained by using a Geiger–Müller tube or a scintillation detector with a circuit which measures the pulse rate.

The energy response of instruments measuring X- or γ-dose rate is important. In Fig. 8.3 typical response curves are shown for the ion chamber, Geiger–Müller tube and scintillation detector. It is seen that the ion chamber has a relatively flat response over the energy region 0.3 to 10 MeV while the response curves for the Geiger–Müller tube and the scintillator tend to peak markedly at low energies. Survey monitors are often calibrated using a radium-226 source, which has an effective photon energy of 0.8 MeV. If the instrument is then used to measure radiation of different photon energy it may seriously underestimate or overestimate the dose rate. Generally, compensating devices are incorporated into instruments using scintillation or Geiger–Müller detectors to give a relatively uniform response from about 0.1 to 3 MeV.

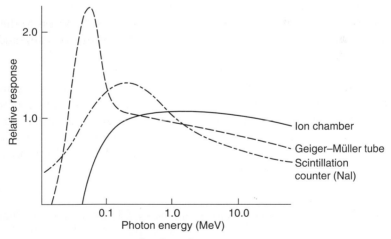

FIGURE 8.3 Energy response curves of various detectors.

A typical survey meter is shown in Fig. 8.4. This is capable of measuring β, X and γ radiation and has a number of advanced features, including automatic range selection and data logging facilities.

8.7.3 Neutron monitors

Neutrons, being uncharged, do not ionize directly and so some indirect means has to be used to produce ionization. Fast neutrons are detected by causing them to interact first

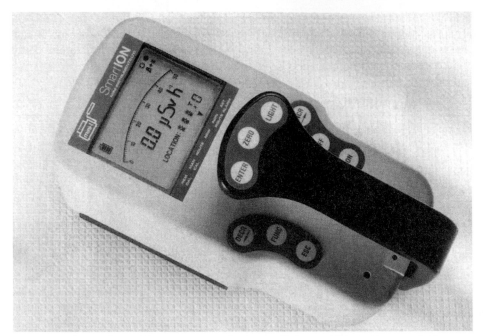

FIGURE 8.4 Advanced portable survey meter (courtesy of Thermo Electron Corporation).

with a material containing a large proportion of hydrogen atoms. The neutrons 'knock-on' protons in the hydrogenous material and the ionization caused by these protons can be detected. Fast neutron monitors often use a proportional counter with some hydrogenous material, such as polythene, incorporated in its volume. These instruments have a very low sensitivity and it is difficult to detect levels below about 50 μSv/h.

The most common reaction used to detect thermal neutrons is:

$$^{10}B(n, \alpha)^7Li$$

Boron-10 has a large cross-section for thermal neutron capture and the emitted α particles cause ionization which may then be detected. The most common thermal neutron monitors employ either an ion chamber lined with a thin layer of boron, or a proportional counter filled with boron trifluoride (BF_3) gas.

The response of instruments using the boron reaction falls off rapidly above energies of a few electronvolts, whereas the instruments using the proton recoil reaction only start to operate at energies above 100 000 electronvolts (0.1 MeV). For many years, there was no instrument that could measure the intermediate energy neutrons which, it is now known, make an appreciable contribution to neutron doses around reactors. However, over the past few decades, instruments have been developed which can measure them.

The emphasis is now on instruments that measure tissue dose over a very wide range of energies from thermal up to about 15 MeV. One such instrument is illustrated in Fig. 8.5. It has a cylinder of polythene which slows down fast neutrons by elastic collisions. A series of cadmium filters are arranged inside the polythene cylinder to give the correct energy response function. The thermal neutrons are detected in a proportional counter filled with helium gas.

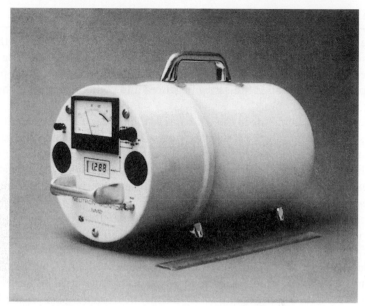

FIGURE 8.5 Neutron monitor (courtesy of Thermo Electron Corporation).

The capture of a neutron results in the emission of a proton according to the reaction:

$$^3He(n, p)^3H$$

where ^3H is the isotope of hydrogen called **tritium**. Once again, ionization is caused by the proton.

This system is now generally preferred to systems using the boron-10 reaction because it is less sensitive to γ radiation.

8.8 PERSONNEL MONITORING EQUIPMENT

8.8.1 Personal dosimetry

Radiation survey monitoring is used to define radiation levels at various points in a laboratory or around a reactor. It is not an accurate method of assessing the accumulated dose received by workers in these areas because:

- it is quite likely that the dose rates will vary considerably with time, depending on the operations being carried out;
- the workers will usually move around from one radiation level to another during the course of their work.

To overcome these difficulties, it is normal practice for people working in radiation areas to wear a **personal dosemeter**. This is a device which measures the dose accumulated by the wearer and there are several types of personal dosemeter in common use.

8.8.2 The film badge

This is the traditional method of personal dosimetry and although methods such as TLD have replaced it to some extent it remains in wide use. The film badge is one of the accepted methods of monitoring whole-body radiation dose for the purpose of record keeping. The developed films may be stored and could, if necessary, be rescrutinized later.

The film badge in general use in the UK consists of a Kodak Personal Monitoring Type 2 film in a special holder. The Kodak Type 2 film is a double emulsion type having a fast emulsion on one side and slow emulsion on the other. The degree of blackening on the developed film is determined using a densitometer and then related by calibration to the radiation exposure of the film. The use of two emulsions permits measurement over a wide range of dose. The fast emulsion enables γ-ray doses in the range 50 μSv to about 50 mSv to be measured. If a dose in excess of about 50 mSv has been received, part of the fast emulsion is stripped from the film and the slow emulsion then permits measurements up to 10 Sv.

The holder is illustrated in Fig. 8.6. It incorporates several filters so that β, γ, X and thermal neutron doses can be measured. Basically, β dose is measured in the open window area, γ dose is measured under the lead and thermal neutron dose is measured by taking the difference between the lead + cadmium and the lead + tin filters. Thermal neutrons interact with cadmium via an (n, γ) reaction and the resulting γ rays give additional blackening under the cadmium filter. The 300 mg/cm^2 and 50 mg/cm^2 filters permit energy

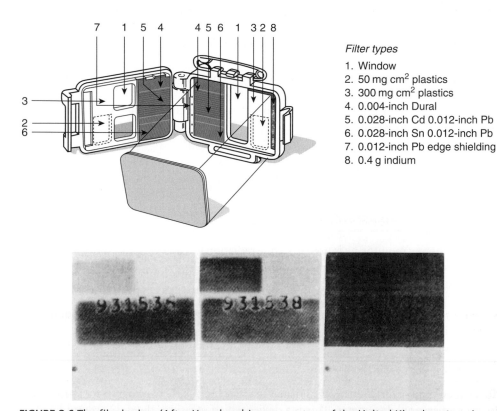

Filter types

1. Window
2. 50 mg cm^2 plastics
3. 300 mg cm^2 plastics
4. 0.004-inch Dural
5. 0.028-inch Cd 0.012-inch Pb
6. 0.028-inch Sn 0.012-inch Pb
7. 0.012-inch Pb edge shielding
8. 0.4 g indium

FIGURE 8.6 The film badge. (After Heard and Jones, courtesy of the United Kingdom Atomic Energy Authority.)

corrections to be applied to the β and low-energy γ doses. The strip of lead around the edge of the holder is to minimize edge effects at the boundary of the various filters. The indium foil is an 'exposure indicator' for criticality accidents. A dose above 10 mSv of thermal neutrons will activate the indium sufficiently to permit measurement using a Geiger–Müller tube.

8.8.3 Thermoluminescent dosemeters

These materials offer an accurate and stable means of measuring dose over the short and long term and find applications both as whole-body and extremity monitors. The action of ionizing radiation on thermoluminescent materials and the method of reading has been described in Chapter 7. One of the disadvantages of this technique is that the process of reading the dose destroys the information, so that, unlike the film badge, the dosemeter can be read only once. The TLD system also provides less information about the quality of the radiation.

Two materials currently in use are lithium fluoride and calcium fluoride. The latter is very sensitive but has a poor energy response. Lithium fluoride is less sensitive but its energy response is excellent. In a practical dosemeter system the thermoluminescent material is usually in the form of a thin disc.

Many establishments are now using TLD systems as the primary method of personal monitoring. This is because they are particularly suitable for automatic linking to computerized dose recording systems. Even in establishments in which the film badge is the main method of personal monitoring, TLD systems are used to provide a convenient method of short-term dose control.

An example of a practical dosemeter system is illustrated in Fig. 8.7.

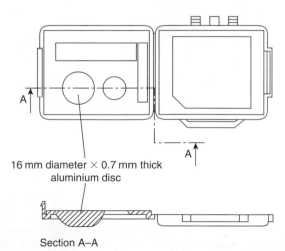

16 mm diameter × 0.7 mm thick aluminium disc

Section A–A

FIGURE 8.7 Thermoluminescent dosemeter (courtesy of the National Radiological Protection Board).

8.8.4 Electronic dosemeter

Various types of electronic dosemeters have been available for some decades, mostly based on miniature Geiger–Müller tubes, providing a direct display of either dose rate or accumulated dose. In many cases, the dosemeters incorporated alarm features to give warning of high dose rate or of reaching a predetermined accumulated dose. Their main application has been to provide an on-the-job method of dose measurement and control.

A new generation of electronic dosemeters has become available, using solid-state detectors and taking advantage of developments in information technology. By means of inbuilt microprocessors and memory they can be programmed to perform a variety of functions, such as logging doses for a specific task or for a shift, or storing information on the characteristics of the radiation field. With gate entry facilities they can be used as a form of security pass, giving recorded access to controlled areas. The devices therefore offer the advantage of combining the operational dose control and the long-term legal dose measurement functions. An example of a modern electronic dosemeter is shown in Fig. 8.8.

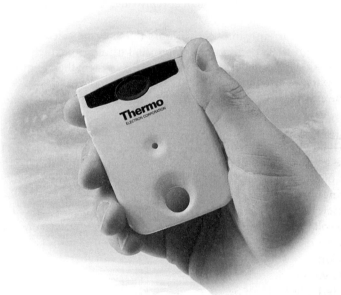

FIGURE 8.8 Commercially available electronic dosemeter (courtesy of Thermo Electron Corporation).

The disadvantages, compared with film dosemeters or TLD, are that they are relatively costly initially, bulky and are potentially susceptible to electromagnetic fields.

8.8.5 Fast neutron dosemeter

The fast neutron dosemeter consists of a nuclear emulsion film sealed in a moisture-proof sachet and worn in a holder similar to a film badge. The holder contains lead, boron and plastic filters to screen the emulsion from body-scattered neutron radiation. The fast neutrons interact with the base material of the film and cause recoil protons to be ejected. These protons create ionization tracks in the emulsion which show up when the film is developed. The tracks are counted under a microscope and the number of tracks per square centimetre is a measure of the neutron dose.

Track plates have a range of 1 mSv to 1 Sv. Their chief drawbacks are that they are expensive to evaluate and have a threshold energy of about 0.5 MeV for detection of neutrons.

In addition, they are sensitive to γ radiation and a dose of about 100 mSv of γ makes the counting of tracks impossible.

8.8.6 Criticality locket

A criticality locket is worn in addition to the film badge or TLD whenever fissile material is handled (e.g. fuel element manufacturing and processing plants, fuel element cooling ponds and reactors). It is designed to measure the very high doses which could be experienced during a criticality accident. The criticality locket contains components which are activated by neutrons of different energies. The reactions utilized in the doseme-ter are:

$$^{32}S(n, p)^{32}P \qquad \text{(S, sulphur; P, phosphorus)}$$

$$^{197}Au(n, \gamma)^{198}Au \qquad \text{(Au, gold)}$$

$$^{115}In(n, n)^{115m}In \qquad \text{(In, indium)}$$

All of the activated components are β-emitters and can be counted in a suitable shielded detection system. From the counts obtained the fast, intermediate and thermal neutron dose can be estimated.

8.8.7 Quartz fibre electrometer

The QFE is a pocket dosemeter, about the size of a large pen, which gives continuous visual indication of accumulated γ dose. It consists of a quartz fibre assembly in a small ion cham-ber, a spring-loaded plunger for charging the electrometer, a microscope lens through which to view the quartz fibre and a scale calibrated in mSv. The electrometer is charged by applying a voltage to the centre electrode which causes the quartz fibre to deflect. When it is exposed to γ radiation the air inside the chamber is ionized and the charge on the electrode reduced. Consequently, the deflection of the quartz fibre is decreased and the change in deflection indicates the dose. Quartz fibre electrometers are available with sensitivities ran-ging from 0–1 mSv to 0–100 Sv.

For many years this device provided a cheap, simple and reliable means of operational dose control but it has now been largely superseded by the new generation of electronic personal dose meters discussed previously in Section 8.8.4.

8.9 RADIATION RECORDS

The purpose of personal dosimetry is to ensure that workers exposed to ionizing radiation are kept within the dose limits specified in the appropriate legislation or code of practice. In most countries, personal monitoring devices other than those for short-term dose control must be provided by an approved laboratory. An approved dosimetry laboratory has the fol-lowing duties:

1. Issue film badges, TLDs and any other personal dosemeters (such as fast neutron track plates) which may be necessary.
2. Process and assess these on return.
3. Issue dose reports and maintain dose records.

Some of the larger employers of workers who wear personal dosimetry devices have established their own processing laboratories. Other users rely on specialist organizations such as, in the UK, the National Radiological Protection Board.

For legal purposes, both film badges and TLD are approved methods of personal dosimetry in the UK. They are normally processed once a month and the results are recorded in the worker's personal dose record. In addition to a monthly dose report, a quarterly summary is normally issued in respect of each employee which summarizes the total radiation dose accumulated over the calendar quarter, year and working life.

As discussed in Section 8.8.4, electronic dosemeters are developing to the extent that they are suitable for use within an approved dosimetry system, although they are not yet widely used for this purpose.

SUMMARY OF CHAPTER

External radiation hazard: arises from radioactive materials outside the body.
Control of external hazard: time, distance and shielding.
Time: Dose = dose rate $\times$ time.
Distance: Inverse square law $D_1 r_1^2 = D_2 r_2^2$.
Dose rate from a γ source

$$D = \frac{ME}{6r^2} \,\mu\text{Sv/h}$$

(M in MBq, E in MeV, r in metres).
Shielding: Alpha particles very easily absorbed.
　　　　　　Beta radiation. Use low Z materials to reduce bremsstrahlung.
　　　　　　Gamma radiation is attenuated exponentially,

$$D_t = D_0 e^{-\mu t}$$

　　　　　　Half-value layer $t_{1/2} = 0.693/\mu$.
　　　　　　Neutron shielding; elastic scatter, inelastic scatter and neutron capture.
Neutron sources: depend on either (α, n) or (γ, n) reactions.
Area classification: uncontrolled, supervised, controlled and restricted areas.
X- and γ-monitors: use ion chambers, Geiger–Müller tubes or scintillation detectors.
Neutron monitors: ideally cover the energy range from thermal up to about 15 MeV, use the reaction $^3\text{He}(n, p)^3\text{H}$ to give good γ rejection.
Personal dosemeters:
　　Film badge, special film with two emulsions to cover range from 50 μSv to 10 Sv, in a holder with filters which allow measurement of β, γ, X and thermal neutron dose.
　　Thermoluminescent dosemeters store the radiation energy which can later be released by heating. The light output is measured using a photomultiplier tube, the electrical output of which is a measure of the radiation dose.
　　Electronic dosemeter: based on solid-state detectors and providing both short-term and long-term measurement capability with direct readout.
　　Fast neutron track plate, special film in a holder, fast neutrons eject recoil protons which cause developable tracks in the emulsion. Main disadvantage is that track plates are expensive to evaluate.

Criticality locket, worn when handling fissile material; the various components are activated by neutrons of different energy and can be counted in a β-castle.

Quartz fibre electrometer, pocket ionization chamber which gives continuous indication of accumulated γ dose.

REVISION QUESTIONS

1. What are the three methods by which the external radiation hazard is controlled?
2. To carry out a certain process a worker has to work in an area which has an average dose rate of 10 μSv/h. How many hours per week can he or she work in this area if 100 μSv/week is not to be exceeded? To what level must the dose rate be reduced to allow work in the area for 40 h/week?
3. Calculate the equivalent dose rate at a distance of 1 m from a 540 MBq cobalt-60 source. At what distance will the equivalent dose rate be 25 μSv/h?
4. The dose rate at a distance of 1 m from a certain γ source is 360 μSv/h. At what distance from the source is the dose rate 10 μSv/h?
5. Calculate the approximate dose rate at a distance of 2 m from a 3000 MBq γ source which emits one 1.6 MeV γ photon per disintegration.
6. Discuss the problem of detecting neutrons and show how it is overcome in modern neutron monitors.
7. List the main types of personal dosemeter and discuss the relative advantages and disadvantages of the film badge, the TLD and the electronic dosemeter.

The internal radiation hazard 9

9.1 UNCONTAINED RADIOACTIVITY

When a radioactive material is enclosed inside some form of sealed container it may give rise to an external radiation hazard to personnel working in its vicinity. Conversely, when radioactive material is not contained in any way it constitutes a potential **internal radiation hazard** and is generally referred to as **contamination**.

Quite small quantities of radioactive material which represent an insignificant external hazard can give rise to appreciable dose rates if they come into contact with, or get inside, the body. Once the radioactive substance is taken into the body it will continue to irradiate the body until either the radioactivity has decayed or the body has excreted the substance. The rate of decay of the radioactivity depends on its half-life, which can vary from a small fraction of a second to many thousands of years. The rate of excretion of the substance from the body depends mainly on its chemical characteristics, and it may happen in a period of a few days or it may take much longer, perhaps many years. Thus, when a radioactive substance enters the body it may irradiate it for only a few days or for a much longer period that may extend to many years in the case of certain nuclides.

9.2 ROUTES OF ENTRY

There are four ways in which contamination can present a hazard to the body. These are:

1. direct **inhalation** of airborne contamination;
2. **ingestion,** that is entry through the mouth;
3. entry through the skin, or through a contaminated wound;
4. direct irradiation of the skin.

When contamination is present in the atmosphere it will be breathed into the lungs and a certain fraction of it will pass into the bloodstream. A fraction of the inhaled contamination will be eliminated from the lungs and swallowed, while the remainder will be exhaled. The various fractions passed into the bloodstream, swallowed or exhaled depend on many factors, such as the chemical and physical form of the contamination, and the metabolism and physiology of the person involved. Similarly, when contamination is ingested, the amount of it passing through the wall of the digestive tract into the body fluids depends on the nature of the contamination and on metabolic and physiological factors.

There are wide variations in the characteristics of human beings and, for the purposes of radiological protection, the International Commission on Radiological Protection (ICRP) defined a **reference man** in *Publication 23*, some of whose characteristics are listed in Table 9.1. It will be seen, for example, that reference man breathes about 23 m^3 of air per day and has a total water intake of 3 litres/day. Reference man is an entirely fictitious individual and simply represents an average over the very wide spectrum of human characteristics.

Table 9.1 Some characteristics of reference man

1. Organs of reference man

Organ	Mass (kg)	Percentage of total body
Total body	70	100
Skeleton	10	14
Muscle	28	40
Fat	13.3	19
Blood	5.5	7.9
Gastrointestinal tract (including contents)	2.2	3.1
Thyroid gland	0.02	0.029

2. Air and water balance

Water intake (litres/day)		Excretion (L/day)	
Foods	0.7	Urine	1.4
Fluids	1.95	Sweat	0.65
Oxidation	0.35	Insensible	0.85
		Faeces	0.1
Total	3.0	Total	3.0

Air balance	
Vital capacity of lungs 4.3 L	
Air inhaled during 8-h working day	9.6 m^3
Air inhaled during 16 h not at work	13.2 m^3
Total	~23 m^3/day

These values are for the adult male. In most cases the values for adult female are lower. For full details of the characteristics of reference man see ICRP *Publication 23*.

In 2003, ICRP published a new Report (*ICRP Publication 89: Basic Anatomical and Physiological Data for Use in Radiation Protection: Reference Values*) which extends and updates the information in *Publication 23*. It moves from the past emphasis on reference man to providing a series of reference values for both male and female subjects of six different ages: newborn, 1 year, 5 years, 10 years, 15 years and adult. Anyone requiring this level of detail should consult *Publication 89*.

It was pointed out above that the fate of a particular radionuclide inside the body depends on its chemical and physical form. For example, some elements distribute themselves fairly uniformly and so irradiate the whole body at about the same rate. The majority of elements, however, tend to concentrate in particular organs so that an intake of radioactivity may result in different dose rates to the various organs of the body. Examples of such elements are iodine, which concentrates in the thyroid gland, and plutonium, which concentrates in the lung or bone.

The dose rate to any organ is proportional to the amount of radioactivity in the organ and decreases as the radioactivity decays or is excreted. The decay of a radionuclide is exponential in character and it is found that the rate of excretion of most substances from the body may also be considered as approximately exponential. This means that an **effective decay constant** can be employed to describe the rate of removal of a radioactive substance from the body (see Fig. 9.1), namely:

$$\lambda_{\text{eff}} = \lambda_r + \lambda_b$$

where

   λ_r = the radioactive decay constant
   λ_b = the biological decay constant.

Since the decay constant is equal to $\log_e 2$/half-life, this equation becomes:

$$\frac{1}{T_{\text{eff}}} = \frac{1}{T_r} + \frac{1}{T_b}$$

where

   T_{eff} = effective half-life of a radioactive substance in the body
   T_r = radioactive half-life of the substance
   T_b = biological half-life of the substance

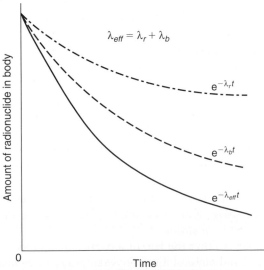

FIGURE 9.1 Typical elimination curve of a radionuclide in the body.

Figure 9.2 illustrates the variation of dose rate with time following an intake of a radionuclide. The initial rise in the curve covers the period during which the nuclide is being transported

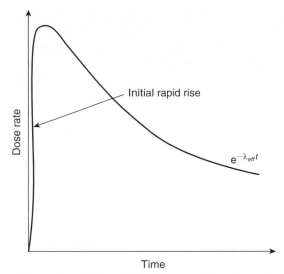

FIGURE 9.2 Variation of dose rate with time following an intake of a radionuclide.

to the organ of interest. At the peak most of the radionuclide that is destined for the particular organ has reached it and the organ is receiving its maximum dose rate. Subsequently, the dose rate to the organ decreases approximately exponentially as the radionuclide decays and is excreted. The total dose received by the organ is obtained by evaluating the area under the curve. Thus a given intake of a radionuclide will 'commit' the organ (or organs) at risk from that nuclide to a certain dose, which is known as the **committed equivalent** dose. This depends on the initial dose rate and on the removal rate. It is usually assumed that a given intake of a particular radionuclide will result in the same committed equivalent dose whether it is received in a single large intake or a large number of small intakes. By applying the tissue weighting factor, the committed equivalent dose can be expressed as a committed effective dose.

For the majority of radionuclides, the dose is received over a relatively short period following an intake, typically a few months to a few years, because after this time the radioactivity will have decayed or have been excreted. For some long-lived species, such as plutonium isotopes, the radioactivity is excreted only very slowly and so the dose is received over a very long period. In this latter case, the committed equivalent dose is defined as that which is received in a period following the intake of 50 years for adults or 70 years for children, as these times represent the likely maximum lifespan of the individual following the intake.

9.3 DOSE PER UNIT INTAKE

Committee 2 of the ICRP, dealing with internal exposure, has calculated values of the committed effective dose for an intake of 1 Bq for virtually all radionuclides that could be of interest in radiation protection. These are referred to as effective dose coefficients for intakes. Separate values are given for intake by inhalation and ingestion. The basic values for adult workers are given in ICRP *Publication 68* and are based on the characteristics of the ICRP reference man from *Publication 23*. Situations can occur in which it is necessary to assess the dose to members of the public, including infants and children, for example where they are exposed to low levels of radioactivity in the environment. The values for members of the public are tabulated in ICRP *Publication 72.*

Table 9.2 illustrates some examples of the dose coefficients for some important radionuclides for inhalation and ingestion. Since the transfer of any material from the lung or from the gut is influenced by its chemical form, particularly its solubility, it is necessary to specify different values for different chemical forms of the majority of radionuclides. It can be seen that the committed effective dose from an intake of 1 Bq varies widely for different radionuclides reflecting the different types of emission (α or β), the half life and the behaviour of the particular chemical form of a radionuclide in the body. Radionuclides with a high dose coefficient are of high radiotoxicity and those with a low value are low radiotoxicity emitters.

Table 9.2 Some values of effective dose coefficient for workers

		Effective dose coefficient, Sv/Bq	
Radionuclide	**Compound**	**Inhalation**	**Ingestion**
Tritium	Tritiated water	1.8×10^{-11}	1.8×10^{-11}
	Organically bound	4.1×10^{-11}	4.2×10^{-11}
	Hydrogen gas	1.8×10^{-15}	–
Sodium 22	All	2.0×10^{-9}	3.2×10^{-9}
Iodine 131	All	1.1×10^{-8}	2.8×10^{-8}
Caesium 137	All	6.7×10^{-9}	1.3×10^{-8}
Plutonium 239	Oxides and hydroxides	3.2×10^{-5}	2.5×10^{-7}
	All other compounds	8.3×10^{-6}	9.0×10^{-9}

These values are for a particle size of 1 μm and are taken from ICRP *Publication 68, Dose Coefficients for Intakes of Radionuclides by Workers, Annals of the ICRP*, **24(4)**, 1994. The corresponding data for members of the public are given in ICRP *Publication 72, Age-dependent Doses to Members of the Public from Intake of Radionuclides: Part 5 – Compilation of Ingestion and Inhalation Dose Coefficients, Annals of the ICRP*, **26(1)**, 1996.

It should be noted that the values recommended by the ICRP are revised periodically in the light of new scientific data and so values from current sources should always be used for radiation protection purposes.

EXAMPLE 9.1

During a particular year it is estimated that a worker has been exposed to intakes of 1.5×10^5 Bq of sodium-22 (via ingestion) and 50 Bq of plutonium-239 oxide (via inhalation). What is the total committed effective dose from the intakes?

For sodium-22, the ingestion dose coefficient (see Table 9.2) is 3.2×10^{-9} Sv/Bq and for plutonium-239 in oxide form the inhalation dose coefficient is 3.2×10^{-5} Sv/Bq.

The committed effective dose from the intakes is then:

For Na-22; 1.5×10^5 Bq $\times$ 3.2×10^{-9} Sv/Bq $= 4.8 \times 10^{-4}$ Sv $= 0.48$ mSv

For Pu-239: 5.0×10^1 Bq $\times$ 3.2×10^{-5} Sv/Bq $= 1.6 \times 10^{-3}$ Sv $= 1.6$ mSv

The total dose is therefore 2.08 mSv.

It should again be emphasized that in radiation protection the primary requirement is not just to maintain doses within the dose limits but to ensure that doses are as low as reasonably achievable within those dose limits. This is particularly important in the case of internal radiation because of the greater difficulty in controlling exposure and of assessing the doses to individuals from intakes of radioactivity.

In assessing the total dose received by a person in a year, both the external and internal doses must be considered to ensure that the recommended dose limit is not exceeded.

9.4 CONTROL OF THE CONTAMINATION HAZARD

9.4.1 Basic principles

As with external radiation, the consideration in the control of the radioactive contamination hazard is to limit the dose to the various organs of the body to the permitted level. However, the basic approaches to controlling exposure are quite different. In the case of external radiation, the dose rate in a working area can be easily measured and the dose received by workers can be continuously monitored and controlled using personal dosemeters. Where there is significant radioactive contamination, however, there is much greater uncertainty both in the levels of radioactivity on surfaces and in the air in the workplace and, particularly, in the quantities likely to be inhaled or ingested by a worker. The approach must therefore be to avoid the contamination of working areas wherever possible and clean up any releases that do occur. In many radioactive facilities there will, nevertheless, be situations where some exposure to contamination is unavoidable, for example, when it is necessary to break into contaminated equipment for repairs or maintenance, and in such situations the approach is to protect the worker by means of appropriate clothing and respiratory protection.

Three basic principles are applied to the control of radioactive contamination:

1. **Minimize** as far as possible the amount of activity being handled.
2. **Contain** radioactive material; normally at least two levels of containment are provided.
3. Follow the **correct procedures** regarding protective clothing, washing and monitoring facilities, etc.

Figure 9.3 illustrates a typical containment system which might be applied in the relatively simple case of a radiochemistry laboratory. The four levels of containment are: the bottle containing the liquid, the splash tray, the fume hood and, finally, the barrier at the entrance to the laboratory.

9.4.2 Area classification

As with the external radiation hazard, routine control of contamination is by means of a system of **area classification**. Table 9.3 shows the basis on which areas should be classified. As can be seen, **supervised areas** are those in which contamination is not normally expected but which could occur due to some failure in equipment or procedures. They provide a useful buffer zone between **controlled areas**, in which contamination is likely to be present to a greater or lesser extent, and uncontrolled areas. Within a controlled area, there could be areas where the contamination hazard is very high and where additional

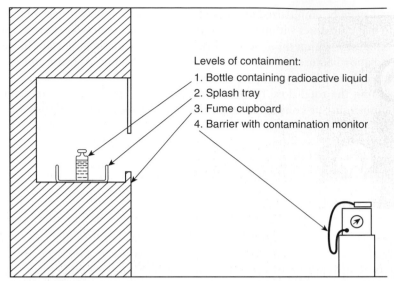

FIGURE 9.3 Schematic diagram illustrating four levels of containment.

Table 9.3 Control levels for area classification

Type of area	Radiological conditions
Uncontrolled (non-active)	No potential for radioactive contamination
Supervised (contamination)	Low potential for contamination but need to keep under review
Controlled (contamination)	Contaminated to greater or lesser extent and requiring appropriate precautions and protection measures

controls are imposed. The essential point is that the system should be designed to provide a safe but practical system of working in the particular conditions.

Whenever possible, contamination should be cleaned up as soon as it occurs. This prevents further spread that makes the eventual decontamination more difficult.

Regular surveys should be made in supervised and controlled areas and in the adjacent uncontrolled areas to ensure that contamination is not spreading beyond the barriers.

9.4.3 Protective clothing

The protective clothing requirements in a contaminated area depend on the nature and amount of the contamination. In supervised areas, where there is a low potential for surface contamination, an ordinary laboratory coat with overshoes and gloves will often be sufficient. In controlled areas, the standard of protective clothing and equipment will be entirely dependent on the conditions. Where there is the potential for airborne contamination, some form of respiratory protection, such as a filter mask or a mask with an air supply, would normally be worn. Where the radioactive contamination is in the form of a contaminated liquid, the worker would normally be required to wear a fully enclosed PVC suit with a filter mask or fresh air supply. Some examples of protective clothing are illustrated in Fig. 9.4.

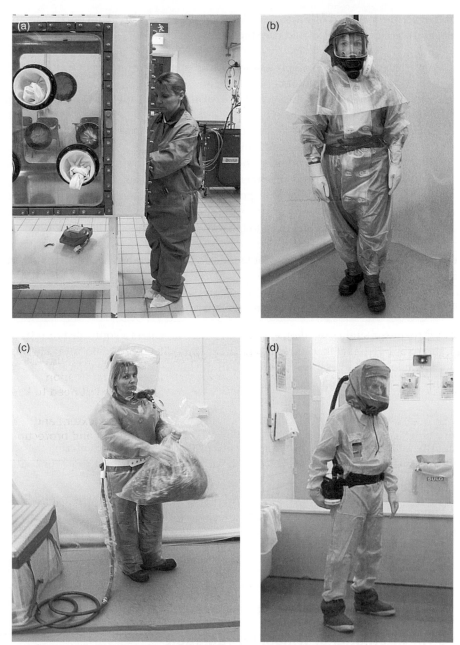

FIGURE 9.4 Protective clothing and equipment. (a) Coverall with gloves and overshoes. Cloth hat would also be worn if required. (b) Impervious clothing and filter respirator. (c) Fully ventilated suit is much more comfortable and more efficient than equipment in (b). (d) Crash suit with self-contained breathing set for emergency use. [(a–c) courtesy of British Nuclear Group, (d) courtesy of British Energy.]

Whatever the standard of protective clothing, the change area and barrier arrangements must be efficient and should have the following facilities:

1. Wash-hand basin (and possibly a shower) and monitoring instruments (for example, a hand and clothing monitor).
2. Suitable stowage on the non-active side of the barrier for the worker's personal clothing.
3. Conveniently placed protective clothing ready for use.
4. Containers for used clothing and radioactive waste.
5. Noticeboards at the barrier stating 'no unauthorized entry', the hazards in the area, the clothing to be worn and any other precautions to be taken.
6. Emergency instructions should be posted in the area, detailing actions in the event of possible incidents such as criticality, fire or serious personal contamination. Consideration must also be given to the provision of suitable emergency exits.

Special arrangements have to be made for laundering clothing worn in contaminated areas and the effluent from laundry facilities is treated as liquid radioactive waste.

9.4.4 House rules and training of personnel

The control of contamination depends on everyone that enters a controlled or restricted area and so all personnel that work in such areas should be given initial and subsequent periodic training in the hazards involved and in the house rules. Some typical house rules for controlled and restricted areas are:

1. No eating, drinking or smoking.
2. No mouth operations (such as pipetting).
3. Any wounds should be covered with waterproof dressing before entering the active area. This is most important since open wounds provide a direct route for contamination into the bloodstream.
4. Wounds sustained in the area should be reported to the person in charge and treated immediately.
5. Ordinary handkerchiefs should not be used in an active area. Disposable tissues should always be available.
6. All items being removed from an active area should be subject to Health Physics clearance before being permitted to leave the area. Active items should be suitably labelled. Whenever possible, sets of tools and cleaning gear should be reserved solely for use in active areas and should be clearly marked as 'active'.

9.4.5 The international symbol for radiation

The internationally agreed symbol for ionizing radiation is the trefoil symbol illustrated in Fig. 9.5. This symbol is found on packages containing radioactive sources, at the entrance to areas where there is a significant radiological hazard, etc.

9.5 RADIOTOXICITY AND LABORATORY CLASSIFICATIONS

A toxicity classification for radionuclides was recommended by the International Atomic Energy Agency (*IAEA Technical Reports Series No. 15*) to act as a guide to the procedures

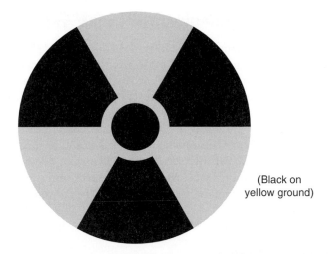

(Black on
yellow ground)

FIGURE 9.5 The trefoil symbol.

and facilities required for handling unsealed radioactive substances. In the classification scheme, radionuclides are divided into four groups according to their radiotoxicity:

Group I – high (e.g. ^{239}Pu and ^{241}Am)
Group II – upper medium (e.g. ^{90}Sr and ^{131}I)
Group III – medium and lower medium (e.g. ^{32}P and ^{65}Zn)
Group IV – low (e.g. ^{129}I, natural uranium)

Note that there are many nuclides in each group and the nuclides mentioned above serve as common examples.

In addition, three classes of laboratory, classes 1, 2 and 3, are defined by the IAEA. A class 1 laboratory is a specially designed facility with elaborate equipment to enable safe handling of high levels of radioactivity. Class 2 laboratories are of a standard comparable to any high-quality chemistry laboratory, whereas class 3 includes ordinary laboratories not originally designed for handling toxic materials. The quantities of radionuclides that can be handled with reasonable safety in the various classes of laboratory are shown in Table 9.4.

Table 9.4 Guide to quantities of radionuclides that may be handled

	Class of laboratory		
Radionuclide toxicity	**3**	**2**	**1**
Group I	Up to 370 kBq	Up to 370 MBq	Above 370 MBq
Group II	Up to 3.7 MBq	Up to 3.7 GBq	Above 3.7 GBq
Group III	Up to 37 MBq	Up to 37 GBq	Above 37 GBq
Group IV	Up to 370 MBq	Up to 370 GBq	Above 370 GBq

These figures are for normal, wet chemical operations. Modifying factors may be applied as follows:

Work	**Modifying factor**
Storage in closed, vented containers	× 100
Simple wet chemistry; low specific activity	× 10
Complex wet or simple dry operations	× 0.1
Dry and dusty operations	× 0.01

9.6 DESIGN OF AREAS FOR RADIOACTIVE WORK

A considerable amount of pre-planning must be done before an active laboratory or active area is set up. Apart from the general features of design expected in any good facility, special attention must be paid to ventilation and to surface finishes. Ventilation systems require efficient filtration units to remove particulate activity before discharge. In the case of gaseous activity, which would not be removed by filtration, great care must be exercised in the location of outlets to ensure adequate dispersal of any discharged activity.

Surfaces in an active area should be smooth and unbroken and be made from materials that are chemically inert, non-absorbent and water-repellent. Consideration must also be given to possible decontamination problems that might arise, and so materials must be chosen which are either easily decontaminated or which can be conveniently removed and replaced.

9.6.1 Walls, floors and ceilings

The basic requirement is that the walls, floors and ceiling should have a good clean finish, free from gaps or cracks in which contamination could accumulate. From the point of view of cleanliness and ease of cleaning it is desirable to have covings at all angles of walls, ceiling and walls, and floors and walls.

Plastered walls and ceilings can be made non-porous and smooth by the application of gloss paint. An alternative approach is to 'face' the walls with a suitable strippable material, for example, melamine laminate on a resin bonded plywood backing which is butt-jointed and the joints sealed. Other finishes that have been used for walls and ceilings include chlorinated rubber-based paint, epoxide resin paint and various other strippable materials.

The most satisfactory floor covering consists of sheet PVC which is stuck down and all joints welded. Such a floor covering should have an integral coved skirting. An alternative covering consists of sheet linoleum which is made water-repellent by applying a hard wax followed by soluble wax. In the case of sheet linoleum a separate preformed coved skirting has to be used and joints have to be cold-welded. PVC or linoleum tiles are not normally recommended because the many joints in the floor make cleaning-up after contamination a difficult operation. Concrete and wood are poor floor materials but their use is sometimes unavoidable. When they have to be used they should be treated with a rubber-based paint to make them water-repellent.

9.6.2 Working surfaces

Working surfaces should be finished in hard non-porous materials which have the necessary heat and chemical resisting properties. The most commonly used materials include:

1. Melamine resin plastic laminate such as Formica. It should be bonded to the backing material with a resin glue to give the necessary temperature resistance.
2. PVC sheet, such as Darvic, which can be welded and is completely self-extinguishing.
3. Stainless steel is a useful material but there is a tendency to get physical bonding between it and corrosion products. Also, stainless steels are susceptible to attack from certain chemicals, for example, hydrochloric acid.
4. Glass fibre reinforced resin which can be moulded to shape. It can be treated to make it fire-resistant, but it may burn in a fire.

5. Polypropylene, which can be welded and heat-formed. This material has such a high chemical resistance that it is difficult to find suitable adhesives for it. It is not fire-resistant and, once ignited, will continue to burn.

9.6.3 Glove boxes

These are installed in active laboratories to facilitate the handling of hazardous materials. They consist of a leak-tight enclosure in which objects or materials may be manipulated through gauntlet gloves attached to ports in the walls of the box (see Fig. 9.6). Their aim is to provide containment for materials that are either radioactive, or chemically toxic, or both. Usually, they do not provide any shielding protection against penetrating radiation and so they are used for α- or β-emitters. When γ-emitting isotopes must be handled, a wall of lead bricks is usually constructed between the operator and the glove box.

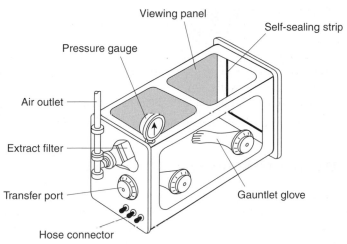

FIGURE 9.6 Schematic drawing of a glove box.

   Glove boxes are maintained at a pressure slightly below that of the outside laboratory. This means that air will flow into the glove box should a leak develop, thus preventing the contamination from escaping. Two filters are normally placed in the ventilation system, one to remove dust from the air being drawn into the glove box and the second to remove radioactive particles from the air being drawn out of the box.

9.6.4 Fume cupboards

A fume cupboard is used when relatively low levels of activity (in the megabecquerel range) are being handled. The material is handled via an opening at the front through which air is drawn from the laboratory into the fume cupboard (see Fig. 9.7). This protects the operator from any leakage of contamination through the opening into the general laboratory. The services usually required in a fume cupboard are water, gas, vacuum and electricity. The controls for these services should be situated outside the fume cupboard to minimize the number of movements through the front opening. It is good practice to ensure that the openings of the fronts of fume cupboards are kept to a minimum to reduce the chance of radioactive contamination entering the general laboratory atmosphere.

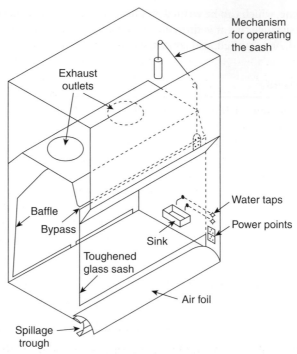

FIGURE 9.7 Schematic drawing of a fume cupboard.

9.7 TREATMENT OF CONTAMINATED PERSONNEL

Once a radioisotope has become lodged in the body, very little can be done to increase the rate of elimination (i.e. decrease the biological half-life) of the isotope. This means that every effort must be made to prevent contamination entering the body. To this end it is vital that all personnel should obey the house rules and always wear the correct protective clothing. Even so, contamination incidents are bound to occur and so a knowledge of the correct treatment is vital.

The first action when dealing with a contaminated person is to ascertain whether or not they are injured. If there is serious injury then first-aid treatment must be given as quickly as possible. Following any necessary medical treatment, the next actions are aimed at removing the contamination before it becomes absorbed and lodged in the body. However, before decontamination can be started, a careful survey must be carried out over the entire body with a suitable contamination monitor to determine the location of the contamination. In the case of partial contamination it is only necessary to decontaminate the affected areas. For example, if a person has received contamination on the hands or face, these areas would be washed thoroughly with soap and water before being monitored again for residual contamination. Should contamination still be present the process is repeated until the affected areas are completely decontaminated.

In the case of whole-body contamination the first action, following removal of protective clothing, would normally be to wash the person's hair over a wash-hand basin. This removes contamination from the hair and prevents it being washed down into the mouth while undergoing whole-body decontamination under a shower using soap or more powerful cleansing agents. After the shower the person is monitored carefully and may need further showers before decontamination is complete. In addition, when the person has been exposed to excessive airborne contamination, other measures, such as nose-blowing and rinsing, may be required to remove the contamination completely.

If a minor wound is sustained in a contaminated area it should be allowed to bleed freely and be copiously washed with water to encourage the removal of the contamination. If the person cannot be immediately and completely decontaminated, or if the wound is serious, medical assistance should be obtained as quickly as possible. When the contamination has been swallowed, substances designed to prevent or reduce absorption from the gastro-intestinal tract, e.g. antacids or ion-exchange resins, may be administered promptly after the intake. If radionuclides of high toxicity, such as ^{239}Pu, are absorbed through a wound or inhaled in a soluble form, certain chemicals called chelating agents may be administered to promote excretion. Unfortunately, these substances tend to be chemically toxic themselves. The absorption of certain radioisotopes can be blocked by the prior ingestion of substantial amounts of a stable isotope of the same element. For example, the uptake of radioiodine to the thyroid can be greatly reduced by previous ingestion of a 200-mg tablet of potassium iodate. This has an important application in the event of a reactor accident.

9.8 CONTAMINATION MONITORING

9.8.1 Sensitivity

It has already been mentioned that quite small quantities of radioactivity which represent an insignificant external hazard can give rise to a significant internal hazard. This means that the radiation levels generated by an amount of radioactive contamination sufficient to cause an internal hazard are generally much lower than the levels that would cause an external radiation hazard. As a result, contamination monitors, in general, need to be more sensitive than radiation survey meters.

To fulfil this requirement for increased sensitivity, contamination meters are constructed from detectors which have their own built-in amplification system (Geiger–Müller or scintillation counters). The activity level is recorded as a counting rate (counts per second or per minute), and the monitor must be appropriately calibrated before the contamination level can be calculated (for example in megabecquerels per square metre).

9.8.2 Direct surface contamination monitoring

This is the simplest and most convenient method of contamination monitoring, and is carried out to establish the presence of contamination on such surfaces as bench tops, clothing, skin and so on. Direct measurements allow the contamination level to be calculated in megabecquerels per square metre, or they can be related to the derived limits of surface contamination. A typical contamination monitor consists of either a mains- or battery-operated ratemeter to which various types of detecting head can be connected.

Alpha contamination is detected by means of a zinc sulphide scintillator coupled to a photomultiplier tube. The zinc sulphide screen is covered with Melinex (DuPont), a very thin plastic material, coated with aluminium to make it light-tight. This covering has to be thin enough to allow α particles to penetrate through to the zinc sulphide screen. It is important when carrying out direct surface monitoring for α contamination to keep the probe as close to the surface as possible to record the true activity level.

Beta contamination monitors usually employ a Geiger–Müller tube in a suitable holder or probe. The probe has a shutter which should be opened for monitoring. If low-energy β

contamination is suspected to be present, a thin end-window Geiger–Müller tube is used. Another type of β detector uses plastic phosphors. These may be used in conjunction with a zinc sulphide screen to form a dual probe which permits simultaneous α- and β-monitoring. A single photomultiplier tube is used with a circuit to differentiate between the α and β pulses.

Beta probes respond to γ radiation, which makes direct contamination monitoring difficult in areas of high γ background. Under such circumstances indirect methods have to be used.

9.8.3   Smear surveys

Smear surveys are an indirect method of measuring surface contamination levels. They are used either to detect very low levels of contamination or to monitor for contamination in an area of high radiation background. A filter paper is wiped over a known surface area (usually $0.1\ m^2$), placed in a polythene envelope to avoid cross-contamination and then taken to an area of low radiation background. Here it is counted in a detecting system of known efficiency. The contamination level can then be calculated from the formula:

$$\text{Contamination level (Bq/m}^2) = C_c \times \frac{100}{E_c} \times \frac{1}{A} \times \frac{100}{E_F}$$

where

C_c = count rate, corrected for background, in counts per second
E_c = overall percentage efficiency of the counting system
A = area smeared in m^2
E_F = percentage of the contamination picked up by the paper.

The last quantity, E_F, is quite difficult to determine and is not very reproducible. It is dependent on various parameters, such as the physical and chemical nature of the contamination, the nature of the base surface, and so on. In some circumstances E_F is taken as 100 per cent and in these cases it is the 'removable' contamination which is being determined. More usually a figure of 10 per cent is assumed.

A useful qualitative technique commonly used within active areas is to swab a large surface area using a damp paper towel and then to monitor the swab. This technique has the advantage that it also decontaminates the surface.

9.8.4 Air monitoring

Air monitoring is carried out in areas where airborne contamination may occur. There are basically three ways by which contamination can become airborne:

1. By disturbance of surface contamination on the surfaces in the active area.
2. By the drying out of liquid contamination.
3. By dry, dusty operations, such as cutting, which cause the release of particulate activity.

Particulate airborne activity is measured by drawing a known volume of air through a filter paper. The filter paper is then counted in a low background area in precisely the same way as for smear survey papers. The level of airborne activity is calculated from the count rate on the filter paper by means of the formula:

$$\text{Airborne contamination level (Bq/m}^3) = C_c \times \frac{100}{E_c} \times \frac{1}{V}$$

where

C_c = corrected count rate in counts per second
E_c = overall percentage efficiency of the counting system
V = volume of air sampled in m^3

Gaseous activity is normally measured by drawing a certain volume of air through a filter paper into a sample chamber, which is then sealed. The filter paper removes particulate activity so that the activity in the sample chamber is caused by radioactive gases only. The chamber is counted in a low background area and the gaseous activity level can be calculated.

9.8.5 Biological monitoring

Normally, airborne and surface contamination monitoring are sufficient to ensure that insignificant amounts of contamination are entering personnel exposed to the contamination. In some circumstances, however, biological monitoring must be carried out. Examples of such circumstances are:

1. The annual limit of intake of the radioisotope in question is very low (for example, plutonium).
2. The isotope is difficult to detect by normal methods.
3. An accident has occurred.

The type of monitoring used will depend on the type of radioisotope inside the body.

Gamma-emitting isotopes can be measured in a whole-body counter, where the subject is placed in a low-background, shielded facility and the γ-emission detected by several large-volume sodium iodide (NaI) scintillation counters.

Alpha- or **β**-emitting isotopes are measured by excretion monitoring, for example, faeces (ingestion of insoluble contamination), urine (soluble contamination). Breath monitoring is carried out to detect the inhalation of radium because radium decays to its gaseous daughter product, radon, which is present in the exhaled breath.

Following a suspected inhalation of activity, monitoring of nasal swabs or nose-blows is a useful indicator of whether or not a significant intake has occurred.

SUMMARY OF CHAPTER

Internal radiation hazard: caused by radioactive materials inside the body.
Routes of entry: inhalation, ingestion and direct entry through wounds in the skin.
Effective decay constant: $\lambda_{\text{eff}} = \lambda_r + \lambda_b$
Committed equivalent dose to an organ: the equivalent dose to which an organ is committed following an intake.
Committed effective dose: the committed equivalent dose to an organ multiplied by the appropriate tissue weighting factor.
Effective dose coefficient: the effective dose from an intake of 1 Bq of a radionuclide. ICRP has tabulated values for all radionuclides of interest for both inhalation and ingestion.
Surface contamination monitoring: direct monitoring, zinc sulphide for alpha detection, Geiger–Müller tubes for β detection. Indirect monitoring using smear surveys.

Surface contamination level:

$$\text{Surface contamination level (Bq/m}^2) = C_c \times \frac{100}{E_c} \times \frac{1}{A} \times \frac{100}{E_F}$$

Airborne contamination level:

particulate contamination level determined by drawing a known volume of air through a filter paper:

$$\text{Contamination level (Bq/m}^3) = C_c \times \frac{100}{E_c} \times \frac{1}{V}$$

gaseous activity measured by drawing a known volume of the atmosphere through a filter paper into a sample chamber and counting the activity.

Biological monitoring:

1. γ-emitters, whole-body counter;
2. α- or β-emitters, faeces, urine or breath monitoring.

REVISION QUESTIONS

1. If a worker is exposed to intakes of 2×10^5 Bq of iodine-131 (via inhalation) and 10^6 Bq of caesium-137 (via inhalation) in 1 year, what is the maximum external dose that he can receive in the year within a 20 mSv annual dose limit? (11.1 mSv.)
2. Calculate the maximum intake of plutonium-239 dioxide which a worker may receive via inhalation in a year if his dose from external exposure is 10 mSv. (312.5 Bq)
3. Discuss the problem of direct surface contamination monitoring.
4. Calculate the surface contamination level from the following data:

Uncorrected count rate on smear paper	3840 counts/min
Background count rate	240 counts/min
Efficiency of counting system	15 per cent
Area of surface smeared	0.1 m^2
Pick-up efficiency of smear	10 per cent

5. Calculate the level of airborne particulate activity from the following data:

Uncorrected count rate on filter paper	29832 counts/4 min
Background count rate	1032 counts/4 min
Efficiency of counting system	12 per cent
Flow rate through particulate sampler	0.03 m^3/min
Time for which sampler was run	2 min

6. Discuss the problem of dealing with a contaminated person who is also injured.
7. What is meant by the 'radiotoxicity' of an isotope? Discuss how this affects the classification of laboratories which handle radioactive material.

Nuclear reactor health physics

10

10.1 INTRODUCTION

The discovery of fission in 1938 provided the basis of a new source of energy potentially greater than the entire world reserves of fossil fuels. The first fission reactor was operated in a converted squash court in Chicago in 1942 by Enrico Fermi and this was followed by a rapid development of nuclear power plants in the 1960s and 1970s. This slowed down in the 1980s and 1990s and many of the early plants are now being decommissioned. However, nuclear energy still supplies a significant fraction of the power requirements of most of the advanced countries of the world.

The advantages of the nuclear reactor as a source of power are offset to some extent by a number of special problems. These include:

1. The protection of the operator and maintainer.
2. The safe treatment and disposal or storage of the radioactivity produced.
3. The need to achieve an acceptably low risk of injury to the public from the potentially large releases of radioactivity that could occur in the event of a reactor accident.

None of these problems is insurmountable and it is generally agreed that, with a small number of exceptions discussed in Chapter 16, the nuclear energy industry has a very good safety record.

To understand the hazards associated with reactors, a basic knowledge of nuclear fission and reactor technology is necessary. In this chapter, after a basic discussion of the process of nuclear fission and of reactor technology, the radiological hazards involved in the operation of nuclear reactors are outlined.

10.2 FISSION

10.2.1 The fission process

Fission is the splitting of a nucleus into two approximately equal parts, known as fission fragments. Certain types of heavy nuclei, notably uranium and thorium, are found to undergo spontaneous fission at a rather low rate. Others can be made to fission by the addition of energy, for example by bombardment with neutrons. Materials which can be made to fission in this way are said to be fissile. The process of fission results in the release of energy, mainly in the form of kinetic energy of the fission fragments. This is rapidly converted into thermal energy and raises the temperature of the fuel material. Of naturally occurring materials, only the isotope uranium-235 (^{235}U) is fissile to a significant extent. This constitutes only 0.7 per cent of natural uranium, the remaining 99.3 per cent being uranium-238.

A fundamentally important feature of fission is that the fission fragments are so unstable that they give off neutrons, usually between two and four neutrons per fission (Fig. 10.1). Most of the neutrons are emitted almost instantaneously, and are called prompt neutrons, but some are released some seconds or even minutes after fission; these are called delayed neutrons.

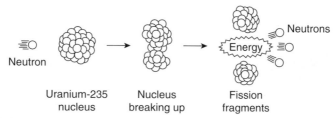

Neutron   Uranium-235   Nucleus   Fission
                 nucleus   breaking up   fragments

Neutrons   Energy

FIGURE 10.1 Fission.

The emission of neutrons by the fission process has a number of consequences. First, it makes possible a chain reaction; second, neutron capture reactions in the uranium fuel result in the production of transuranic elements, including plutonium (see Section 10.2.4); and third, neutron captures in the structural and other materials of nuclear reactor plants result in these materials becoming activated (see Section 10.2.5).

10.2.2 Chain reactions and criticality

The neutrons emitted after fission may themselves cause further fission with the emission of more neutrons, so making possible a chain reaction. In practice some of the neutrons escape from the system and others are captured in non-fission reactions. In a reactor, wastage of neutrons by capture reactions is minimized by taking care to exclude materials of high capture cross-section from the core. Some loss is inevitable since even the fuel material can capture neutrons without fission. By increasing the size of the core the fraction of neutrons escaping can be reduced to a sufficiently low level to permit a chain reaction. If a core is very small, neutrons can easily escape but in larger cores they would require to travel further and are, therefore, more likely to cause fission. Another method of reducing leakage is to put a reflector of some light material around the core to reflect escaping neutrons back into the core.

Consider an assembly of fissile material in which, on average, 2.3 neutrons are produced by each fission. If, on average, 1.3 neutrons are lost by leakage or capture, one neutron is available to cause a further fission. This results in a self-sustaining chain reaction in which the fission rate is constant. Such a system is said to be **critical**. An average loss of 1.31 neutrons for every fission means that only 2.3 − 1.31 = 0.99 neutrons are available for fission. The system is then subcritical and the fission rate will decrease. Conversely, for a loss of 1.29 neutrons per fission, 1.01 neutrons remain. This results in a supercritical system in which the fission rate will increase.

Thus, for any given type of reactor there is a minimum size of core below which the system cannot go critical. Alternatively, a certain minimum mass of fuel is required for a chain reaction to be possible; this is the minimum **critical mass**. For example, a nuclear weapon can, in principle, be made from two pieces of fissile material each of which is slightly more than one half of the critical mass. The weapon is detonated by bringing the two pieces rapidly together to give a supercritical mass. This results in the fission rate, and hence the rate of energy release, rising very rapidly to enormous values. Fortunately, this is rather difficult to achieve in practice.

The possibility that fissile material could 'go critical' if assembled in a sufficient quantity has very important implications in the design and operation of plants in which it is processed, handled or stored. It is obviously very important to ensure that criticality does not occur and this is usually achieved by careful design of the facilities supplemented, in some cases, by operational procedures. This aspect is discussed further in Chapter 16.

10.2.3 Fission products

In fission, the splitting of the atoms of a fissile material can occur in many different ways. The most likely division of the heavy atom is into fragments of mass about 97 and 135. For example,

$$^{235}_{92}U + ^{1}_{0}n \longrightarrow ^{135}_{52}Te + ^{97}_{40}Zr + 4^{1}_{0}n$$

The distribution of mass number of fission products is of the form shown in Fig. 10.2. The fission process produces about 300 different nuclides, most of which are neutron-rich and decay by a series of β-emissions through a decay chain of radioactive nuclides. In the example of fission shown above, tellurium-135 and zirconium-97 both undergo a series of β-decays until a stable nuclide is produced:

$$^{135}_{52}Te \longrightarrow ^{135}_{53}I \longrightarrow ^{135}_{54}Xe \longrightarrow ^{135}_{55}Cs \longrightarrow ^{135}_{56}Ba$$

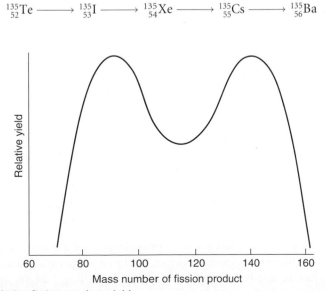

FIGURE 10.2 Relative fission product yield.

and

$$\ce{^{97}_{40}Zr} \longrightarrow \ce{^{97}_{41}Nb} \longrightarrow \ce{^{97}_{42}Mo}$$

It will be seen that the utilization of nuclear fission to produce energy results in the formation, within the fuel, of hundreds of different types of radioactive fission products with half-lives varying from a fraction of a second to very many years. The inventory of fission products in the fuel builds up over the period of irradiation.

Figure 10.3 shows the fission product inventory, in becquerels, and its decay from 1 to 1000 days in fuel which has produced a uniform 1 MW of heat over a 2000-day irradiation.

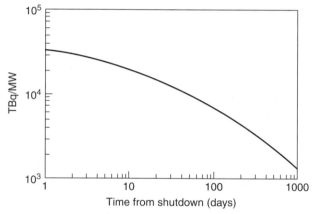

FIGURE 10.3 Approximate fission product β inventory in fuel, irradiated for 2000 days at 1 MW.

The many different nuclides present as fission products have a very wide range of physical and chemical properties and so the radiotoxicity of the different nuclides varies enormously. To prevent the fission products escaping, the fuel is contained within another material of suitable properties, known as the **fuel cladding**.

10.2.4 Transuranic elements

As previously noted, neutrons can be captured by fuel atoms in non-fission reactions. Successive capture reactions and β-decays result in the generation in the fuel material of transuranic elements, that is, elements higher in the periodic table than uranium. Of particular importance is neutron capture in ^{238}U, yielding ^{239}U, which quickly undergoes β-decay to neptunium-239 (^{239}Np), and then to plutonium-239 (^{239}Pu).

$$\ce{^{238}_{92}U(n, \gamma)^{239}_{92}U} \xrightarrow{\beta} \ce{^{239}_{93}Np} \xrightarrow{\beta} \ce{^{239}_{94}Pu}$$

This is a process of great importance since it provides a route whereby a large proportion of ^{238}U, which is not fissile to a significant extent, can be converted into ^{239}Pu, which is fissile. However, ^{239}Pu has the disadvantage of being a long-lived ($T_{1/2}$ = 24 300 years) α-emitter and, unlike uranium, it is of very high radiotoxicity.

Further capture and β-decay processes lead to the production of americium (Am) and curium (Cm) nuclides.

10.2.5   Activation products

Neutron capture in structural materials and in the coolant of a reactor results in the generation of many species of radioactivation products. In steel components, the stable iron isotope ^{58}Fe undergoes neutron capture to become ^{59}Fe, which decays by β-emission to cobalt-59 (^{59}Co) with a half-life of 45 days.

In many cases, because of a particular combination of nuclear properties, activation of trace elements in a material is important. For example, all types of steel contain cobalt, normally at a concentration of only a few hundred parts per million. The stable isotope ^{59}Co is activated by the reaction

$$^{59}\text{Co} \, (n, \gamma)^{60}\text{Co}$$

Cobalt-60 has a relatively long half-life of 5.22 years and, in addition to a low-energy β particle, emits two energetic γ-rays per disintegration.

In both water-cooled and gas-cooled reactors, an important reaction on the oxygen component of the coolant is

$$^{16}\text{O}(n, p)^{16}\text{N}$$

Although nitrogen-16 has a very short half-life of 7.2 s, it has a great influence on the shielding requirements for all reactors.

10.3 REACTOR SYSTEMS

10.3.1 General features

The great majority of commercial nuclear power reactors currently operating or under construction, worldwide, are light water reactors (LWR), which were originally developed in the USA. These are of two types, pressurized water reactors (PWR) and boiling water reactors (BWR). In a PWR a closed water coolant system transfers heat from the core to heat exchangers, which raises steam in a secondary circuit to drive a turbogenerator (see Fig. 10.4). In a BWR, the water passing through the core is allowed to boil and the steam is passed directly to the turbines. Another type of water-cooled reactor is the Canadian CANDU system which uses heavy water as the neutron moderator.

In the UK, a different line of development was pursued and resulted in two generations of gas-cooled reactors. In the earlier type, known as the Magnox reactor, the core consists of a very large graphite structure, penetrated by channels containing natural uranium fuel rods clad in a magnesium alloy and cooled by carbon dioxide. The carbon dioxide circulates through heat exchangers, where steam is raised as in a PWR. The second-generation UK plants are known as advanced gas-cooled reactors (AGR). To achieve a higher operating temperature, stainless steel fuel cladding is used and this necessitates the use of enriched uranium, as discussed in the following section. Typical Magnox and PWR plants are illustrated in Figs 10.5 and 10.6 (page 106).

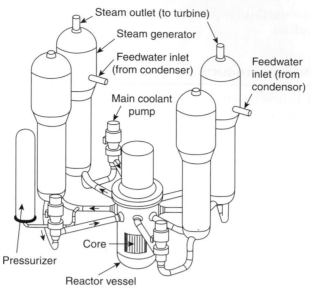

FIGURE 10.4 Primary system of a pressurized water reactor.

Another system is the sodium-cooled fast breeder reactor, sometimes known as the liquid-metal fast breeder reactor (LMFBR). The original concept was that fast reactors would use plutonium fuel extracted from spent thermal reactor fuel but, later, would breed enough plutonium by neutron capture in ^{238}U in and around the core to meet their own fuel requirements. The development of fast reactors has slowed down considerably because of difficult engineering problems leading to significantly increased cost, and also because the expected scarcity of uranium has not materialized.

More recently, there has been renewed interest in the high-temperature gas-cooled reactor (HTGR) which uses helium gas to cool ceramic uranium fuel. In one design, (known as the Pebble Bed Reactor), the fuel consists of many thousands of ceramic spheres, through which the helium passes to remove the heat. The temperature of the helium gas as it exits the core is much higher than in existing gas-cooled reactors and so a direct turbine cycle should theoretically be possible. However, HTGRs present a number of novel radiological challenges.

The central features of any nuclear reactor are: the core, which contains the fissile material; a means of controlling the fission rate; and a moderator in the case of thermal reactors but not in the case of fast reactors. The other main features are a cooling system to remove the heat generated by fission and a radiation shield, often called the biological shield. These various features are described below.

10.3.2 The core and control system

The reactor core contains fuel elements which consist of fissile material in a fuel can or covered by a cladding material which prevents the escape of the fission products. The fuel is normally uranium although plutonium and thorium are sometimes used. Naturally occurring uranium contains 0.7 per cent of the isotope ^{235}U and 99.3 per cent of ^{238}U. Magnox and CANDU systems are able to operate using natural uranium, but in other

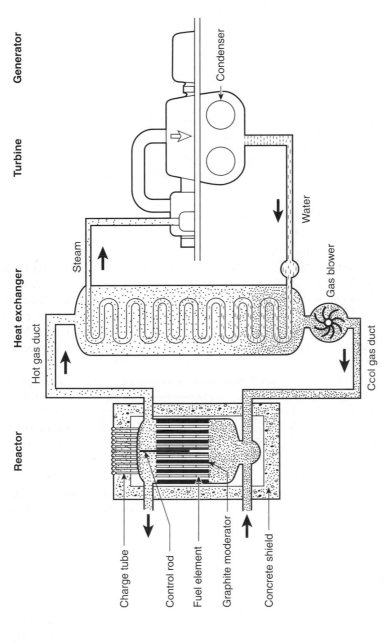

FIGURE 10.5 Schematic illustration of a Magnox power reactor.

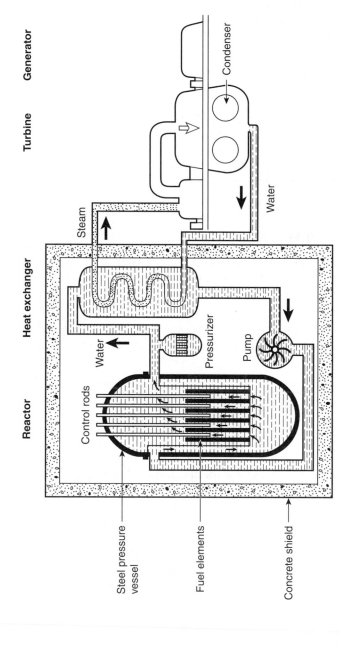

FIGURE 10.6 Schematic illustration of a pressurized water reactor.

systems it is necessary to use uranium containing a higher percentage of ^{235}U and this is achieved by means of an enrichment process.

The moderator serves to slow down the fast neutrons produced by fission to the thermal energy range in which they are most likely to cause further fission. In light water reactor systems, the water serves both as moderator and coolant, while in the gas-cooled systems the moderator is graphite.

The control rods are made from materials of high neutron absorption cross-section such as boron or cadmium. Withdrawal of the control rods to a certain minimum position takes the reactor critical. Further withdrawal makes the reactor supercritical and the fission rate increases. When the required power is reached, insertion of the rods to the critical position causes the power to become constant. The reactor power can be reduced by insertion of the rods to a subcritical position. The control system is based on a number of neutron detectors around the core. If the neutron flux exceeds a preset value or if it is increasing too rapidly the detectors sense it and the reactor is automatically shut down by the rapid insertion of the control rods (or sometimes special shut-down rods). Various other monitoring systems provide data which can shut down the reactor if something goes wrong; for example, by detecting high γ radiation levels outside the biological shield, excessive core or coolant temperature, or loss of coolant flow.

10.3.3 The cooling system

Fission causes energy release within the fuel and consequent temperature rise of the fuel and cladding material. The heat is removed by the coolant and steam is raised, directly or indirectly, to drive turbines. Various subsidiary systems are provided for coolant purification, sampling and so on.

The integrity of the cooling system must be very high. Most coolants become radioactive to some extent and even small leaks may pose radioactive contamination problems. Large leaks could limit the heat removal from the core and affect the safety of the reactor. It is important to realize that in a power reactor the decay of the fission products generates a substantial amount of heat and so cooling must be guaranteed even when the reactor is shut down.

10.3.4 The biological shield

The purpose of the biological shield is to attenuate the neutron and γ radiation from the reactor core and cooling system so that the operators and maintenance staff do not receive excessive doses. The most commonly used materials are lead, concrete, iron, water and polythene. In the case of power reactors the factor of reduction required may be of the order of 10^8 to 10^9. Weaknesses can arise in the shield where coolant ducts and other penetrations offer streaming paths for radiation. The shield is often constructed in two parts: the primary shield around the reactor core and the secondary shield around the cooling system. This arrangement permits access to the coolant system (circulators, heat exchangers, etc.) when the reactor is shut down since the γ radiation from the decay of fission products is attenuated by the primary shield.

10.4 REFUELLING REACTORS

In a nuclear reactor, 1 kg of natural uranium (occupying a volume of about 50 cm^3) can produce as much energy as 10 tonnes of coal burned in a conventional power station.

This is despite the fact that only 0.3 per cent of the uranium atoms are burned up, which represents about 40 per cent of the fissile ^{235}U atoms. The percentage of uranium which can be burned up is limited, since a stage is eventually reached when insufficient fissile material remains to sustain the chain reaction. In addition, pressures generated by the fission products in the fuel cause swelling and distortion of the fuel elements. When a fuel element reaches the required burn-up, it must be removed from the reactor (remember that it is intensely radioactive), and replaced by a fresh element.

In the large gas-cooled reactors, refuelling of the reactor is often performed with the reactor operating. The operation is performed by a remotely controlled charge/discharge machine on top of the reactor which removes the shielding plug, seals itself on to the pressure vessel and removes the fuel channel cap. The spent fuel elements are raised from the channel into the machine, which is heavily shielded, and replaced by fresh elements. When the machine contains its full quota of elements it is moved to a position where the elements can be released through a shielded chute into a large tank of water, known as a cooling pond, which provides shielding and cooling for the spent elements. The machine is designed so that these operations can be carried out safely. It must, therefore, provide shielding from the reactor core above the unplugged hole, provide shielding from the spent fuel elements inside the machine, prevent leakage of gas or contamination and provide cooling for the fuel elements (the heat generated by decay of the fission products in an element when it is removed from the reactor is sufficient to cause it to overheat unless external cooling is provided).

In LWR, on-load fuelling is not possible for a number of reasons and refuelling is performed during the annual shutdown when about one-third of the core is replaced. This involves flooding a canal above the reactor pressure vessel, removing the pressure vessel lid and lifting the fuel elements out one at a time into the water-filled cavity. They are then transferred down the canal into a storage pond.

10.5 RADIATION HAZARDS FROM REACTORS

10.5.1 General

In general, reactors are a lesser radiation hazard when they are operating than when they are shut down. The shielding is designed to give acceptable radiation levels at working positions and this is confirmed by thorough surveys during the commissioning of the plant and subsequently at regular intervals. Systems are provided which permit safe means of sampling coolants and other radioactive effluents. During shut-down periods, a great variety of non-routine jobs may be undertaken, some of them on highly radioactive systems. It is during such periods that exposure of personnel to radiation and radioactive contamination must be carefully controlled.

A serious fault or maloperation could cause considerable damage to the plant and give rise to dangerously high levels of radiation or radioactive contamination. If the hazard is confined to the reactor site it is often called a site emergency but if it extends off-site it may become a public emergency. Accidents of this type are discussed in Chapter 16.

10.5.2 Sources of radiation

The main sources of radiation from a reactor at power are the core and the coolant. The radiation from the core includes fission neutrons, fission γ-rays, fission product decay

γ-rays, neutron capture γ-rays and activation product decay γ-rays. The last two arise predominantly in the core structure and shield. The radiation from the coolant is mainly γ-rays arising from activation of the coolant, activation of impurities and fission product contamination of the coolant. The sources are illustrated in Fig. 10.7.

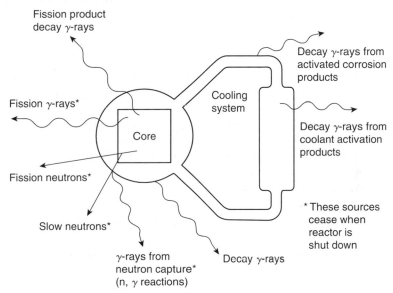

FIGURE 10.7 Sources of radiation in a nuclear reactor system.

RADIATION FROM THE CORE

The neutrons produced in a reactor as a result of the fission process are fast neutrons in the range of 0.1–15 MeV, average energy about 2 MeV. Those emerging from the surface of the biological shield have undergone varying degrees of moderation and so neutrons of all energies from thermal to fast may be present.

Fission γ-rays are those emitted immediately after the fission fragments and vary in energy from 0.25 to about 7 MeV. The γ radiation resulting from the decay of fission products in the fuel elements is small compared with the fission γ radiation but, whereas the latter ceases on shutdown of the reactor, the fission products continue to emit radiation for many years after the fuel has been withdrawn from the reactor.

Neutron capture in the structural materials of the reactor and in the shield results in the emission of capture γ-rays and makes these materials radioactive. The radiation from the decay of the radioactivity, as in the case of fission products, continues to be emitted when the reactor is shut down. Neutron scattering also leads to γ-ray emission but does not, in general, induce radioactivity.

RADIATION FROM THE COOLANT

As noted previously, in both water-cooled and carbon dioxide-cooled reactors, the reaction

$$^{16}O(n, p)^{16}N$$

is important because nitrogen-16 decays with a half-life of 7.2 s and emits very penetrating (6.1 MeV) γ-rays. This means that the coolant circuit of the reactor is a significant source of γ radiation and, in most cases, must be shielded.

Air was used as a coolant in a number of reactors of early design and is used on Magnox reactors to cool the biological shield. Air is also present as an impurity in the coolants of both gas- and water-cooled reactors. The argon which is present to the extent of 1.3 per cent in air is activated by the reaction:

$$^{40}Ar(n, \gamma)^{41}Ar$$

Argon-41 decays with a half-life of 1.8 h and emits γ radiation of energy 1.29 MeV.

In LMFBR, which use sodium as a coolant, the important activation products are sodium-22 (^{22}Na) and sodium-24 (^{24}Na).

Although reactor coolants are very pure by normal standards, there are always some impurities. When subject to the very high neutron flux in the reactor core, these impurities become radioactive to an appreciable extent. Impurities also arise as a result of corrosion or erosion from the core and the coolant system. For example, in Magnox and advanced gas-cooled reactors, graphite dust (which itself contains impurities) collects around the cooling system. In water-cooled reactors, iron, nickel, cobalt and manganese are common impurities because of corrosion of the coolant system. Deposition of this corrosion material in the core causes the build up of a film of corrosion products on fuel surfaces. As a result of irradiation by neutrons, these films become highly radioactive. The continuous release of material from the core and subsequent deposition in the out-of-core regions causes a build-up of radioactivity in the coolant system.

Reactor coolants usually contain readily detectable levels of fission product contamination arising from:

1. Uranium contamination on the fuel element surface.
2. Uranium impurity in the fuel cladding material.
3. Release from a damaged fuel element.

The coolant is being continually cleaned up by a treatment system and so the long-lived fission products do not build up appreciably. The predominant fission product activities are usually krypton-88 (^{88}Kr) and xenon-138 (^{138}Xe) which are inert gases, their particulate daughter products rubidium-88 (^{88}Rb) and caesium-138 (^{138}Cs), and the three isotopes of iodine, ^{131}I, ^{133}I and ^{135}I. A seriously damaged fuel element could lead to a considerable fission product activity being spread around the cooling system. Most gas-cooled reactors are fitted with a system known as 'burst can detection' which continuously and automatically 'sniffs' each channel in turn and gives warning to the operators if an increase in the fission product activity should occur. The channel containing the damaged fuel can is then unloaded and the faulty element is replaced. In water-cooled reactors, the presence of fission products in the coolant is detected by radiochemical analysis.

10.5.3 Sources of radioactive contamination

BETA EMITTERS

Almost all of the radioactive nuclides mentioned in the preceding paragraphs decay by β-emission. Beta radiation is so easily absorbed that the shielding designer does not even need to consider it, concentrating instead on the associated γ-emission. On the other hand, if radioactive contamination occurs, owing to a leak of radioactivity from the reactor system, the β radiation is often of prime importance.

A radionuclide of considerable importance which is produced in all reactor systems is tritium (^{3}H). This nuclide has a half-life of 12.3 years and decays by low-energy β-emission only. It is produced by fission, by a (n, γ) reaction on deuterium (hydrogen-2), and by various reactions on lithium and boron. In reactors cooled or moderated by heavy water, large amounts of tritium build up. In light water systems, because of the much lower concentration of deuterium and the frequency of water change (heavy water is much too expensive to change), build up of tritium is usually less significant. Lithium and boron are present in most systems, either as additives, neutron absorbers or impurities, and can contribute to tritium production by a number of reactions, including:

$$^6\text{Li}(n, \alpha)^3\text{H and } ^{10}\text{B}(n, 2\alpha)^3\text{H}$$

COOLANT LEAKS

Contamination can, of course, occur because of a coolant leak. In pressurized water systems the leak may be direct to the atmosphere or via a heat exchanger into the secondary system, in which case radioactivity, mainly the gaseous activities ^{88}Kr, ^{138}Xe and ^{41}Ar, would be carried over with the steam into the turbines and then to the atmosphere via the condenser air ejector. The fission product gases ^{88}Kr and ^{138}Xe decay to their particulate daughters ^{88}Rb and ^{138}Cs. A leak in the heat exchanger of a gas-cooled reactor would normally cause steam to leak into the primary system because of the higher secondary pressure.

CONTAINMENT

The core of a reactor at power contains about 0.2 TBq of fission products per watt of thermal power. Thus a reactor operating at, say, 1000 MW contains about 2×10^8 TBq of fission products. This vast inventory of radioactivity is contained within the fuel can or cladding, which provides the first level of containment. The second level of containment is the boundary of the primary systems, that is, the pressure vessel and the coolant system. This boundary also contains the radioactivity of the coolant which, in a 1000-MW reactor, may amount to some hundreds of terabecquerels. Provided that the primary and secondary containments remain intact there is little risk of serious contamination. In practice, some contamination does occur during the operation of most reactors. For example, it is usually necessary to sample the coolant periodically and there is often some radioactive effluent. A contamination hazard could arise in both cases but the risk is minimized by good design of facilities.

In its most common usage, the term 'reactor containment' refers to the structure within which the whole system is housed. The function of this containment is to protect the general public by limiting the release of fission products in the event of a serious reactor accident (see Chapter 16).

10.5.4 The shut-down reactor

MAINTENANCE

A reactor represents a large capital investment and shut-down periods, whether scheduled or not, are costly. Reactor systems are comparatively simple, well engineered and normally very reliable. The majority of maintenance, either corrective or preventive, is on ancillary or secondary equipment. A major overhaul may include decontamination and refitting of coolant circulators, control rod mechanisms, inspection of heat exchangers and various other jobs on radioactive systems. At such times, the need to keep to a tight schedule can lead to a general reduction in standards of safety, both radiation and conventional, because it may slow down the work. To prevent this state of affairs, all major work must be planned in consultation with interested parties and sometimes it is desirable to rehearse particularly difficult jobs. Personnel should receive instruction in general safety matters and be familiar with the particular hazards associated with their own work.

EXTERNAL RADIATION

When the reactor is shut down, the primary shield gives adequate protection against the fission products in the core. The radiation hazard to personnel working on the primary system is caused by radioactivity within the system. The dose rate in the vicinity of the primary system tends to decay rapidly in the first 24 h after shut-down, mainly because of decay of coolant activities or their clean-up by the treatment system. Thereafter, the levels do not change significantly from day to day. The half-lives of most of the radioactive corrosion products are in the range of 1 month to about 5 years. The dose rates vary considerably from reactor to reactor but in systems with corrosion problems, levels of 10–100 mSv/h can be encountered on certain components. If the dose rate is excessive it is sometimes possible to provide additional shielding on 'hot-spots'. An alternative approach is to decontaminate the component but this would only be done during major shut-down periods.

Careful control is required of personnel working in areas of high dose rate. This often takes the form of a manned control point at the entrance to the area. Personnel entering the area are given a 'working time' based on a radiation survey of the area. In addition to their normal film badge they are required to wear some form of direct reading dosimeter such as an electronic dosimeter. The times of entry and exit and the dosimeter reading are logged.

CONTAMINATION

When maintenance involves breach of the primary coolant system, contamination is likely to occur. When first breaching part of the system it is obviously essential to have depressurized it. It is good practice for the personnel involved to wear full-face masks when first breaking into any part of the system.

The standards of protective clothing required are evaluated from experience on a particular plant. There are often other factors such as temperature, humidity and possible presence of toxic gases, all of which affect the choice of protective clothing and equipment. Personnel cannot be expected to wear impervious clothing, such as PVC suits, in temperatures of 40–50°C, unless the suits are fully ventilated. This in turn causes difficulties in confined spaces because of the required air-lines. Efficient changing and monitoring facilities are essential. If significant levels of contamination are present, it is advisable to have an attendant to assist in the removal of contaminated clothing. This can often be the same person who logs the entry of personnel.

Frequent monitoring of levels of contamination both inside and outside the area is undertaken to ensure proper control.

10.6 RESEARCH REACTORS

Research reactors, of which there are many different types, present special health physics problems. The reactors have a wide range of applications, including fundamental research, materials testing and the commercial production of radioactive sources. The main radiological problems usually arise, not from the reactor, but from the experimental equipment. For example, there are often holes through the shielding to obtain high-intensity beams of neutrons outside the reactor for various purposes. Rigs containing experimental equipment or materials become highly radioactive. In these and other situations special precautions are necessary to protect both operators and users of the reactor.

10.7 FUEL STORAGE PONDS

10.7.1 Introduction

After removal from a reactor, it is usual to allow the fuel to decay for some months in a fuel cooling pond situated close to the reactor. This procedure eases some of the problems involved in moving the highly radioactive fuel from the reactor site to the fuel reprocessing plant or storage facility. In addition to the routine operational problems, ponds pose two special hazards: criticality and loss of shielding accidents.

10.7.2 Criticality

Ponds often contain enough fissile material to 'go critical', that is, to initiate a fission chain reaction. In general, if only natural uranium fuel is in the pond criticality is not possible even under the worst possible conditions. If enriched uranium or other fissile material such as plutonium is present, criticality could conceivably occur. The hazard is controlled by storage in safe configurations, that is, with adequate spacing between fuel elements or by limiting the number of elements which may be out of their storage position at any time.

10.7.3 Loss of shielding

A typical storage pond may often contain thousands of terabecquerels of fission product activity and a single element may contain a few hundred terabecquerels. Such an element unshielded would give a γ dose rate in excess of 1 Sv/h at a distance of 3 m. Obviously, this situation must not be allowed to occur. Loss of shielding can occur by loss of pond water or by raising fuel too close to the surface of the water. Loss of pond water is more likely to result from accidental pumping out rather than from a leak caused by serious structural damage. The possibility of pumping out can be minimized by a good design of the water system and by administrative control of the system (e.g. locks on vital valves).

It is difficult to safeguard completely against a fuel handling accident without defeating the advantages of water shielding, such as visibility and flexibility. Good design of lifting tackle can make it impossible to raise fuel too high but only if the correct tackle is used. A little ingenuity can defeat the best systems. Considerable reliance is placed on installed γ monitors to give warning of potentially dangerous situations.

10.7.4 Operational aspects

The fission product activity of the fuel is contained within the fuel cladding. A breach of the cladding would lead to contamination of the water by fission products to some extent, depending on the form of the fuel. As a precaution against the release of gaseous fission products, which would be rapidly released from the water surface, many ponds have an air extract system 'sweeping' the water surface. Some degree of water contamination also occurs as a result of the release of radioactive corrosion products from the surface of the fuel cladding. To prevent build-up of activity a water treatment system is provided. A water cooler is usually necessary, depending on the amount of fuel stored.

Cutting operations in a pond can lead to serious contamination problems from swarf, particularly if fuel is cut. The maintenance of the cutting equipment may be hindered by high contamination and radiation levels.

10.7.5 Pond instrumentation

There are three main types of instrument used to give warning of hazardous conditions:

1. Installed γ monitors are an essential feature of any fuel storage pond. At least three instruments are necessary and they should be situated so that they cannot be shielded from the pond surface. A local alarm such as a bell or buzzer should sound if any of the instruments reaches some quite low level, say 0.1 mSv/h. This would warn the operators that a potentially dangerous situation is developing. At some higher radiation level, say 10 mSv/h at the **operator's position** an evacuation alarm should sound. This alarm should operate on a two out of three or two out of four basis to avoid spurious evacuations.
2. Pond water counter: this is a simple device which continuously monitors the water for β activity and gives early warning of damaged fuel. A shielded liquid flow Geiger–Müller tube connected to a ratemeter is often used.
3. Air monitor: a continuously operating airborne particle monitor in the general area or in the air extract gives warning of high airborne contamination arising from pond operations or maintenance of pond equipment.

10.8 FUEL REPROCESSING

After a period of pond storage at the reactor site to allow some decay of the levels of radioactivity and decay heat, irradiated fuel may be transported to a fuel reprocessing plant. Here, after a further period of pond storage, the fuel is dissolved in nitric acid and the solution is chemically separated into three main streams: unused uranium, plutonium and a highly active waste stream containing almost all of the fission products and higher actinides such as americium and curium.

A reprocessing plant poses much greater radiological problems than a reactor because of the nature of the processes involved. Essentially, a reprocessing plant is a complex chemical facility, processing intensely radioactive solutions that must be shielded from operating areas by 1 m or more of concrete. This plant requires maintenance and, although facilities are provided to enable much of it to be done remotely, some contact maintenance is inevitable. Although the part of the plant requiring maintenance will have been decontaminated, this is never completely effective. In addition, relatively small leaks of the radioactive solutions into the shielded 'cells' of the plant cause severe radiation and contamination problems, and decontamination of cell and equipment surfaces is very difficult and time-consuming.

Of the product streams, the uranium stream does not present any significant radiological problem, but the plutonium stream demands extremely high standards of containment to avoid a severe contamination hazard, particularly through inhalation.

In addition to the highly active waste stream, which is routed initially into special storage tanks, there are a number of subsidiary radioactive waste streams, the treatments of which depend on local conditions. The management of radioactive waste is covered in Chapter 11.

Another important factor in the design and operation of fuel cycle facilities is the possibility of a criticality accident. Such an accident could result not only in high neutron and γ radiation from the event, but also, because of the energy generated, in dispersal of the process material.

10.9 DECOMMISSIONING OF REDUNDANT NUCLEAR FACILITIES

With many of the first-generation nuclear research and power-generation facilities now closed down, the decommissioning of redundant nuclear plant has become a major issue in the safety, economics and environmental impact of the nuclear industry. The early plants were constructed without any consideration of the eventual need for their decommissioning and, in many cases, this has necessitated complex and expensive approaches. In later plants, the need to make suitable design provision to facilitate decommissioning was recognized and this is expected to yield both radiological and economic benefits in the longer term.

The special problems that arise in dealing with redundant nuclear facilities arise from the radioactivity remaining in the plant at the end of its useful life. This has three technical implications:

- a high standard of containment of the radioactivity is needed in order to protect the local population;
- the residual radioactivity in the plant poses a radiological hazard to workers involved in the decommissioning of the plant; and
- the radioactive structures and equipment are important sources of radioactive waste streams, both directly and because of the secondary wastes that arise from decontamination and dismantling operations.

The key to a successful decommissioning project is preplanning and this normally commences some years before the scheduled closure. The first steps are to prepare a detailed inventory of the plant, equipment and structures, and a full radiological characterization. The characterization is based on a detailed programme of measurements, supplemented, in most cases, by calculations. This allows the radioactive inventory of the many different components of the plant to be estimated. It also permits estimates to be made of the radiological hazards associated with dismantling operations in order to provide a basis for selection of the most suitable engineering approaches. For example, where the assessment shows that very high radiation levels would be encountered, consideration would need to be given to the use of remotely operated equipment. The radiological characterization also allows estimates to be made of waste arisings and of the types of packages needed.

From a radiological point of view, the aim of a decommissioning programme is the progressive reduction of the hazard posed by the plant. For this reason, the first stage of decommissioning is a general clean-up of the facility and the removal of process materials and wastes. The nature of the tasks involved is often similar to those encountered during operation. In the case of a reactor, the major activity at this stage is the defuelling of the core and the removal of fuel from the site. This removes a large proportion of the radioactive inventory and essentially eliminates the possibility of a major release. For process plants, the first stage would be a postoperational clean-out of process equipment, often referred to as a POCO, to remove as much as possible of the process material. The next stage would normally include the removal of auxiliary plant and equipment, particularly those items that are not radioactive and are not needed to support the decommissioning operations.

Beyond this stage, the approach adopted for any particular facility depends on a number of factors, including the radioactive inventory and its pattern of decay, and the relative costs of different options. There are important differences of principle involved in the decommissioning of reactors compared with fuel cycle facilities or other radioactive plant. In particular, the residual radioactivity in a reactor is almost entirely in the form of activated structural materials while in other plants the radioactivity is in the form of process residues and general contamination of plant structures and equipment. Thus, decontamination of a reactor system, although often a useful step, might not significantly reduce the overall radioactive inventory or the radiological impact of dismantling the plant. In other types of plant, early decontamination is a key factor in relation both to exposure of personnel and the management of radioactive waste. Another difference is the pattern of decay of the radioactivity. In the case of a reactor, the activation product cobalt-60 (half-life 5.2 years) usually dominates the inventory, and so substantial benefits, in the form of reduced operator exposure and lower waste arisings, can be gained by delaying the dismantling for a few decades. In fuel plants, little advantage accrues from such a delay because of the long half-lives of many of the radionuclides present in the plant.

The nature of decommissioning operations requires a high level of health physics surveillance. During dismantling of equipment and structures, there is always the potential for an unexpected radiological hazard resulting from, for example, a release of contamination or loss of shielding of a radiation source. Regardless of how well the plant has been characterized in advance, events such as this can occur and this means that radiological conditions need to be continuously monitored during dismantling operations. Levels of worker exposure also need to monitored continuously, preferably by electronic dosimeters that give a direct readout. The standards of protective clothing and equipment worn by workers need to be kept under review. Certain operations might require full respiratory protection but if this requirement is applied excessively, the result could be to slow down operations and increase the dose from external radiation. Although projects are undertaken within a strict management regime using a predefined and approved methodology, it is important that the management and approval regime is sufficiently flexible to be able to take advantage of lessons learned as the project proceeds.

Another important aspect of decommissioning concerns the release of land on which there has been a nuclear or other form of radioactive facility. Even after the plant and structures have been removed, there is always the possibility that low levels of radioactivity will remain on or under the surface of the site. Before such a site can be released for other use, it is necessary to go through a formal monitoring and clearance process. The monitoring involves a detailed programme of both direct radiation monitoring and of soil sampling for laboratory analysis. Where significant levels of site contamination are detected, a programme of site remediation must be undertaken. This might entail the excavation of areas of the site and removal of the soil to a suitable approved landfill site. In other cases, depending on the levels and extent of the contamination, the radionuclides present and the planned use of the site, it may be acceptable to bury the contaminated soil directly on the site, ensuring that there is an adequate thickness of cover. The criteria for clearance of sites vary to some extent from country to country. For clearance of nuclear sites in the UK, the regulatory authority considers that any residual radioactivity above the natural background that can be demonstrated to pose a risk to any person of less than one in a million per year would be broadly acceptable. This corresponds to an average radiation dose-rate above that from natural background of about 20 μSv/year.

SUMMARY OF CHAPTER

Fission: splitting of nucleus into two fission fragments which decay to fission products. Neutron chain reaction requires a critical mass.

Reactor system: the core consists of fissile material, control rods and moderator; other important features are the cooling system and the biological shield.

Refuelling: on- or off-load, depending on the reactor type.

Sources of radiation when operating: fission neutrons and γ-rays, fission product decay γ-rays, neutron capture γ-rays and activation product decay γ-rays.

Shut-down sources: fission and activation product decay γ-rays.

Contamination: may occur owing to coolant leak or maintenance operations.

Containment of fission products is vital to prevent overexposures.

Fuel storage ponds: two special hazards; loss of shielding and criticality.

Fuel reprocessing plant: chemical separation of fuel into uranium, plutonium and waste streams. Severe radiological problems.

Decommissioning: the dismantling of plant, equipment and structures at the end of the useful life of a facility; the importance of preplanning; first stage is initial clean-up and, in reactors, removal of fuel; timing of later stages depends on type of plant.

Remediation: the clean-up and clearance for other use of a site on which there has been a radioactive facility. Needs very detailed survey of radiation and contamination levels and may require removal of contaminated soils and rubble to a special disposal site. Clearance criteria based on risk.

REVISION QUESTIONS

1. Describe the process of nuclear fission and explain the circumstances under which a fission chain reaction may be achieved.
2. Draw a simple sketch of a typical nuclear reactor and label the major features of the system.
3. Using a simple diagram, illustrate the sources of radiation from a nuclear reactor system, indicating which are important when:
   (a) operating;
   (b) shut down.
4. What is meant by containment in the context of nuclear reactors?
5. Discuss the main hazards presented by fuel storage ponds and how they are controlled.
6. What is a fuel reprocessing plant and what are the main radiological hazards encountered?
7. Discuss the factors that could affect the timing of the decommissioning programmes for nuclear reactors and other types of radioactive plant.

Radioactive waste

11.1 INTRODUCTION

Before the discovery of nuclear fission and its utilization as a source of energy, the disposal of radioactive waste did not present a significant problem. It has been estimated that the total quantity of radioactivity in use in research and medicine in 1938 was less than 30 TBq, corresponding to about 1 kg of radium derived from natural sources. Today, a single large power-generating reactor may contain in excess of 10^8 TBq of fission products and there are several hundred power reactors in the world. With the increasing emphasis on protection of the environment, the management of these wastes is becoming an important factor in both the economics and the public acceptability of nuclear power.

On a much smaller scale, radioactive wastes arise in hospitals, factories, research facilities and teaching institutions as the result of a wide range of applications of radiation. In such cases, the complex treatment plants used at nuclear power stations would be prohibitively expensive and so simpler disposal methods are used which might even be via the normal refuse collection or sewage systems. Clearly, the consequences of all such practices must be understood and strict control exercised.

Radioactivity cannot be destroyed. It will decay eventually but, in view of the very long half-life of many radionuclides, it is not always practicable to await the decay of radioactive material. There are three general approaches to the management of radioactive wastes:

1. **release** and **dispersal** into the environment;
2. **storage**; and
3. **disposal**.

Of course, release of radioactivity to the environment might reasonably be thought to constitute disposal. However, it is useful to distinguish between deliberate dispersal and methods of disposal involving irretrievable placement of wastes so that they are isolated, at least temporarily, from the environment.

Storage of radioactive waste is a particularly useful procedure when dealing with nuclides of relatively short half-life (e.g. up to a few months). Storage or hold-up of the waste for a period of up to a few years may reduce the activity to a sufficiently low level to permit release to the environment or, in the case of solid waste, to facilitate disposal.

The approach selected in a given situation depends on many factors, such as the quantity and type of radioactivity, its physical and chemical forms and the geographical location.

In this chapter, after a discussion of the consequences of release of radioactivity, the application of these alternative approaches to the management of liquid, gaseous and solid wastes is discussed.

11.2 CONSEQUENCES OF RELEASES OF RADIOACTIVITY

Any release of radioactivity is a potential source of radiation exposure to the population at large. The radiation exposure can occur via many different **exposure pathways**. Consider, for example, a release of activity from a chimney stack. This would be dispersed by air movements and could result in radiation exposure of the population in a number of ways:

1. Direct external β or γ radiation from the plume.
2. Inhalation of radioactivity resulting in internal dose.
3. Direct external β or γ radiation from deposition (fall-out) of radioactivity.
4. Consumption of foodstuffs (e.g. vegetables) contaminated by deposition.
5. Consumption of meat or milk from animals which have grazed on contaminated ground.

Similarly, radioactivity discharged into a river, lake or sea could result in human exposure via a number of pathways, such as:

1. Contamination of drinking water supplies.
2. External dose to swimmers or to people using contaminated beaches.
3. Consumption of contaminated fish, shellfish or plants.

Some of these exposure pathways result from complex routes known as **food chains**. For example, activity discharged to the sea may be taken up by plankton which are eaten by fish, which are in turn eaten by Man. An example of a simple marine food chain is illustrated in Fig. 11.1.

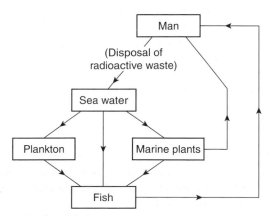

FIGURE 11.1 A simple marine food chain.

In a given situation it is often found that one particular pathway is much more important than any other. That is, it results in much more radiation dose, sometimes to quite a small group of people. This is called the **critical exposure pathway** and the group of people that receives the highest dose from this pathway is known as the **critical group**. The importance of identifying the critical exposure pathway is that it allows the quantity of radioactivity discharged to be controlled so as to limit the dose to the critical group. The critical group in any particular case depends on the mode of release, the nuclides involved, local ecology (e.g. forms of marine life, etc.) and local habits.

The fuel reprocessing plant at Sellafield, in the UK, provides a classic example of the application of this concept. In the plant, irradiated fuel from reactors is processed chemically to recover uranium and plutonium. The other elements, including the fission products and higher actinides, which are intensely radioactive, are transferred to special storage facilities (see Section 11.5). However, a small proportion of the activity appears in subsidiary waste streams, which, after a period of storage to permit some decay, are discharged into the Irish Sea.

Before any activity was released from the plant a detailed study was made to estimate how much activity could safely be discharged. This involved investigations of the local tidal currents and the dispersion that would occur, and of the local ecology. This preoperational study suggested that there would be three main exposure pathways and these involved deposition of activity on sand and silt, uptake in fish and uptake of activity in a variety of edible seaweed. It was anticipated that the last pathway would be the most important and this was subsequently confirmed when the plant became fully operational. This pathway arises because one of the fission products, ruthenium-106 (^{106}Ru), is taken up very efficiently and effectively reconcentrated by the seaweed *Porphyra umbilicalis*. At that time this seaweed was harvested on the coast close to Sellafield and was used to produce a foodstuff called **laver bread** which is consumed in South Wales. Thus the factor which controlled discharges from the plant was the dose from ^{106}Ru to the gastrointestinal tract of laver bread consumers. Later, harvesting of *Porphyra* ceased and the emphasis shifted to the other pathways, including plutonium in winkles and caesium in fish.

The significance of deposition of activity on sand and silt is that beaches and estuaries become contaminated and this leads to external radiation exposure of people using the beaches and of fishermen, for example, when handling nets and equipment. Resuspension of activity into the atmosphere when the beaches dry out has been identified as a possible exposure pathway, as was transfer from the sea via sea-spray into the atmosphere and then onto land. This could be of particular importance in the case of relatively small quantities of plutonium and other actinides.

The activity taken up by fish is primarily caesium-137 (^{137}Cs). Because the caesium is soluble in sea water and because of its 30-year half-life, it disperses over a very wide area giving a low but measurable concentration not only in the Irish Sea but also in the North Sea and even in the Norwegian Sea. This leads to low but measurable concentrations of the activity in fish caught over a very wide area. One important point that emerged from experience at Sellafield is that when long-lived activity such as plutonium is released into the environment it could give rise to a continuing radiological impact.

Recently, the levels of discharge have been considerably reduced and the radiological impact is low for all of the exposure pathways.

In the case of discharges to atmosphere, an important exposure route is the uptake of radioiodine, mainly iodine-131 (^{131}I), in the thyroid as a result of releases of fission products to the atmosphere. The uptake may be from inhalation of airborne iodine or consumption of milk from cows that have grazed on contaminated pasture. In either case, exposed children comprise the critical group because of the relatively large intake by children in proportion to the size of the thyroid.

In all of these cases, the discharge limits are set to be as low as reasonably achievable, so that the critical group receives doses well below the permissible level.

11.3 RADIOACTIVE LIQUID WASTE

Various approaches are used in the management of radioactive liquid wastes. Where the level of radioactivity is very low, liquid wastes can often be discharged either as a trade waste to sewers or directly into a river or lake, or into coastal waters. As discussed earlier, a period of storage might be necessary or worthwhile to allow the decay of relatively short-lived radio-nuclides. In this case, a number of delay tanks would be provided and when one became full it would be isolated until the activity had decayed to an acceptable level for release. Before discharge, the contents of the tank would be stirred, sampled and analysed to confirm that it is within the prescribed activity limits.

Liquid wastes of higher specific activity may be treated by ion-exchange, evaporation or chemical treatment, followed by filtration. These processes result in the concentration of the radioactivity from the liquid waste into a much smaller volume of residue or sludge, which may be suitable for conversion into a solid waste for storage or disposal. The effluent from the process would normally be of sufficiently low activity to permit its discharge.

Discharge to sewers is a very convenient method for hospitals, research institutions and other facilities, where both the volume and specific activity are low, but it is strictly controlled. The main considerations are that sewage, sewer walls and sewage works become contaminated, resulting in a hazard to sewage workers. In addition, sewage sludge is often used as a fertilizer and, if it is contaminated, could result in contamination of crops.

Discharge of radioactivity into rivers is limited by the subsequent use of the river water. Most major European rivers are sources of drinking water and of water for irrigation of crops and watering of cattle. These considerations mean that discharges into most rivers are limited to quantities of the order of a terabecquerel per year, the actual quantity depending on local conditions. Similarly, in the case of lakes, the restricted dispersion usually limits the allowable discharge rates of most nuclides to relatively low levels, again typically a few terabecquerels per year.

In principle, relatively large quantities of radioactivity can be discharged into the sea provided that steps are taken to ensure adequate dilution and dispersal. The limits are usually dictated by food chains involving reconcentration effects in marine organisms as described in Section 11.2. At most coastal locations, discharges of some hundreds of terabecquerels would be possible without leading to excessive dose to the critical group. However, discharge of radioactivity into the environment is a very contentious issue and the emphasis is on ensuring that discharges, and hence critical group doses, are as low as reasonably achievable. The Convention for the Protection of the Marine Environment of the North-east Atlantic (known as the OSPAR Convention), to which the European Union (EU) is a signatory, has set the objective of preventing pollution of the maritime area from ionizing radiation through progressive and substantial reductions of discharges, emissions and losses of radioactive substances, with the ultimate aim of concentrations in the environment near background values for naturally occurring radioactive substances and close to zero for artificial radioactive substances. In effect, this removes discharge into the sea as a significant waste management option.

Whatever the mode of liquid discharge, authorizations need to be kept under continuous review and the safety of the procedure confirmed by environmental monitoring programmes. In the case of marine discharges, this should include measurements on sea-water, fish, seaweed and the seashore and seabed.

11.4 RADIOACTIVE GASEOUS WASTE

Releases of gaseous or airborne particulate radioactivity to the atmosphere present more direct exposure pathways than other forms of disposal and, with a few exceptions such as the noble gases, the discharge limits are quite low. The exposure pathways include external irradiation, inhalation and ingestion by various routes (see Section 11.2). The general philosophy is to reduce the activity being released to atmosphere as far as practicable and then to release it in such a way as to obtain adequate dispersal.

The methods available in practice to achieve these objectives are:

1. Filtration to remove particulate activity.
2. Scrubbing or adsorption systems to reduce gaseous activity.
3. Dispersal via a chimney stack.

Filtration is a very common method and is usually incorporated in extracts from any area containing significant activity. The efficiency of the filter depends on the size of the particles but is usually better than 99.9 per cent. It must be remembered that the filters become radioactive and when they are changed they must be handled with care and treated as solid radioactive waste. Scrubber units and adsorption beds are bulky and expensive items and are used only in large installations such as nuclear reactor plants.

When relatively small amounts of activity are involved the releases to the atmosphere are usually from an extract discharging at, or even below, roof level. Care must be taken in the siting of such extracts since, under certain weather conditions, eddies and currents may cause the released activity to re-enter the building through air intakes or even through open windows. A chimney stack is preferable but the additional cost is only justifiable when large quantities of activity are being released. Ideally, the chimney should be two to three times the height of surrounding buildings to obtain good dispersal. This is illustrated in Fig. 11.2 which shows the dispersion from (a) a short stack and (b) a tall stack on a large building. Even with the tall stack, diffusion or spreading of the plume means that at some distance downwind the concentration of activity at ground level will show an increase. The maximum concentration usually occurs at a distance downwind of 10–20 times the height of the stack, depending on wind and weather.

As with liquid wastes, the adequacy of controls is confirmed by detailed environmental monitoring programmes.

11.5 RADIOACTIVE SOLID WASTE

Radioactive solid wastes arise in various forms in nuclear facilities and from medical and industrial applications of radioactivity. They are usually considered to fall into three broad classes: **low, intermediate-** and **high-level** wastes.

Low-level waste (LLW) consists typically of general trash from contaminated areas as well as items of lightly contaminated or activated plant and equipment. Intermediate-level wastes (ILW) arise mainly in nuclear facilities and include solidified process residues and significantly activated items. The definitions of LLW and ILW, in terms of specific activity,

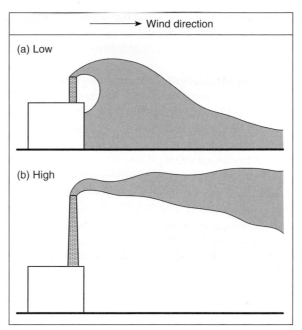

FIGURE 11.2 Dispersion from chimney stacks.

vary from country to country but, typically, LLW would comprise waste of less than about $10^9\,Bq/m^3$ and ILW would be any waste, other than high-level waste (HLW) as defined below, exceeding this value. With both LLW and ILW, disposal is often facilitated by segregation of the waste, preferably at the point of arising, for example into wastes of different specific activity, or into combustible and non-combustible material. Reduction of volume is usually beneficial and this can be achieved either by compaction of the waste or, in the case of combustible waste, by incineration. In the latter case, the fuel gases from the incinerator are normally filtered and the filters and ash then comprise the reduced volume of waste.

The term HLW is usually reserved for the raffinate from the first extraction cycle in a fuel reprocessing plant. This stream contains 99 per cent or more of the fission product activity from spent nuclear fuel and much of the α-emitting higher actinides. The specific activity of this waste is so high that it generates significant heat, and special provision has to be made for cooling. Initially, the waste is stored as a liquid in high-integrity tanks with multiple cooling systems and located inside massive concrete-shielded cells. After a delay of a few years to allow some of the shorter-lived activity to decay, the waste is vitrified, which means that it is incorporated into large glass blocks in stainless steel canisters. The waste is then in a suitable form for safe storage for an extended period.

Storage can only be regarded as a temporary solution to the problem of managing radioactive waste. This is because many types of waste contain long-lived radioactivity. For example, the activity in HLW includes the fission products strontium-90 and caesium-137 with half-lives of 28 and 30 years, respectively. After about 500 years these will have decayed to negligible levels but significant amounts of longer-lived nuclides will remain, including the α-emitters americium-241 (^{241}Am, half-life 434 years), plutonium-239 (^{239}Pu, half-life 24 000 years) and neptunium-237 (^{237}Np, half-life 2.2 million years).

The need to establish safe methods of radioactive waste disposal is an important factor in the public acceptance of nuclear power. In some countries, further development of nuclear power has been made dependent on establishing the feasibility of the safe disposal of wastes.

A method practised by smaller users of radioactive materials, such as hospitals, universities and industrial users, is disposal with ordinary trade waste. The principle being applied here is **dilution**, the odd package containing a small quantity of radioactivity being well diluted and buried among the vast quantities of ordinary trade and domestic waste on the local refuse tip. This approach requires very strict control and the quantity per package is usually limited to about 0.1 MBq.

For the much larger volumes and higher radioactive concentrations of wastes arising from the nuclear industry, two types of special disposal facilities, or waste repositories as they are known, are in use or planned. The first is a shallow land facility in the form of a large engineered concrete structure 10–30 m below the surface, usually in clay beds. This type of repository is suitable mainly for LLW, but may also be suitable for short-lived ILW.

The second type is a deep underground disposal facility, perhaps about 300 m or more below the surface. During the emplacement phase such facilities would be similar to mine workings, with shafts and tunnels. The wastes, contained in high-integrity packages, would be placed in tunnels which would then be back-filled with absorbent materials and, eventually, the workings and shafts would be completely sealed. This type of repository is potentially suitable for both ILW and HLW.

The important consideration in underground disposal is that the waste containment will eventually be lost and activity will be leached into groundwater, though this could take thousands or even hundreds of thousands of years. This could result in the contamination of drinking water supplies or of crops. Disposal sites must be carefully selected to minimize these effects. Another consideration, particularly for shallow land sites, is the possibility of inadvertent human intrusion at some future time. Examples of intrusion are drilling of boreholes, tunnelling and excavation. While controls over the development of the site should be able to ensure that intrusion does not occur for some hundreds of years, beyond this time it is not possible to guarantee that intrusion would not occur. For this reason, the amount of long-lived waste placed in shallow land repositories will need to be strictly limited.

11.6 REGULATIONS

The legislation and regulations covering the management and disposal of radioactive waste vary from country to country. Within the EU, member states implement the Basic Safety Standards Directive in national legislation. For example, in the UK, those aspects of the Directive relating to radioactive waste are implemented mainly through the provisions of the Radioactive Substances Act (1993).

The majority of small users of radioactive sources are required to register the use and storage of radioactivity with the Environment Agency, under the provisions of the Act. Authorizations for disposal are granted by the Agency after consultation with others, including local authorities.

Operators of nuclear installations such as nuclear power stations, fuel manufacturing and reprocessing plants are exempted from the requirement to register their use and storage of radioactive materials. Instead, they are subject to the provisions of the Nuclear Installations Act (1965), (1969) and amendments. In the latter Act reference is made to the

Radioactive Substances Act and the responsibility for authorizing discharges again rests with the Environment Agency. In Scotland the responsibility for authorizing discharges rests with the Scottish Environment Protection Agency.

SUMMARY OF CHAPTER

Main sources of radioactive waste are reactors and the use of radioisotopes in medicine, industry and research.

Principles applied are release and dispersal, storage and disposal.

Consequences of disposal: dose to population via exposure pathways; direct or via food chains. The emphasis is on ensuring that the doses received from waste disposal operations are as low as reasonably achievable.

Limiting pathway is the critical exposure pathway, and population group receiving highest dose is critical group.

Liquid waste: low-level liquid wastes discharged to environment. High specific-activity wastes treated by ion-exchange, evaporation or chemical treatment.

Gaseous waste: release to atmosphere after filtration or scrubbing. Discharge from stack to achieve good dispersal.

Solid waste: LLW, ILW and HLW. Storage is only a temporary solution for long-lived wastes. Segregation and volume reduction facilitate disposal. Possible routes are shallow or deep underground disposal.

Regulations: authorization is required for storage or disposal of radioactive waste.

REVISION QUESTIONS

1. List the three general approaches for dealing with radioactive waste. Give a practical example in each case.
2. Discuss the concept of critical exposure pathway and give an example of such a pathway which involves a food chain.
3. What are the alternative discharge routes for low-level liquid waste? Discuss the factors which limit the quantities that may be discharged in each case.
4. What are the possible exposure pathways resulting from releases of radioactivity to the atmosphere? How would the exposure from these pathways be limited?
5. Discuss the possible disposal routes for radioactive waste. Broadly, what types of wastes are suitable for each route?

X-rays and radiography

12.1 INTRODUCTION

X-rays were discovered in 1895 by the German physicist Wilhelm Conrad Roentgen. During the course of experiments on electrical discharge tubes he noticed that a screen coated with barium platinocyanide glowed when placed near the tube. After further investigation he concluded that the fluorescence was being caused by invisible rays that were capable of penetrating not only glass but also optically opaque materials. He also found that he could photograph the interior of objects. For example the bone structure of the hand could be photographed because the bone attenuates X-rays to a greater extent than the soft flesh. Photographs obtained by passing X-rays through objects (or people) in this way are known as **radiographs**. The medical implications of this discovery were immediately appreciated and, within a few months, physicians in many parts of the world were using X-rays as an aid to diagnosis. These physicians became known as **radiologists** and, as mentioned in Chapter 5, many of them died as a result of excessive exposure to radiation. X-rays are now widely used in medicine, not only for diagnosis but also for the treatment of diseases. They also have applications in industry and in research.

Like light, radio waves and γ-rays, X-rays belong to the electromagnetic group of radiations. They have no mass or charge, but have a wavelength which depends on their energy. They differ from γ-rays in two important respects. First, γ-rays originate within atomic nuclei whereas X-rays originate from changes in the electron orbits. Second, γ-rays from a given source have definite discrete energies but X-rays usually have a broad range or spectrum of energies up to some characteristic maximum value.

The most important method of producing X-rays depends on a process known as **bremsstrahlung** which is German for **braking radiation**. Bremsstrahlung X-rays are produced when charged particles, usually electrons, moving with a very high velocity are slowed down rapidly by striking a target. For example, when β radiation from a radioactive source impinges on a shielding material, bremsstrahlung is produced. The efficiency of X-ray production by this means is dependent on the atomic number (Z) of the target material, high-Z materials giving a much higher yield than low-Z materials. (This is the reason for using low-Z materials such as Perspex for shielding beta sources.) In any case the intensity of X-rays produced by β-particles is too low for most applications. The method used to produce X-rays for medical and industrial purposes uses an electrical discharge tube and is similar to the method used by Roentgen, though modern equipment is much safer and more efficient.

12.2 X-RAY EQUIPMENT

12.2.1 General

X-rays are produced when electrons moving with high velocity are suddenly stopped by a material of high atomic number, and so an X-ray generator requires a source of electrons, a means of accelerating them to a high velocity and a target at which they are directed. An X-ray set consists of a tube and various electrical circuits which are usually in a separate control unit.

12.2.2 Hot cathode X-ray tubes

The modern type of X-ray tube, illustrated in Fig. 12.1, consists of a cathode and an anode inside a glass tube evacuated to an extremely low pressure. The cathode is the source of the electrons and consists of a tungsten filament heated to incandescence by an electric current which 'boils out' electrons. The electrons are accelerated to the target by a high voltage applied between the anode and cathode.

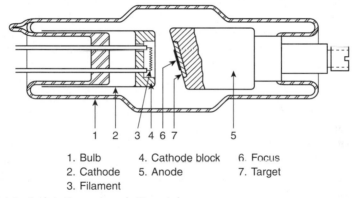

1. Bulb   4. Cathode block   6. Focus
2. Cathode   5. Anode   7. Target
3. Filament

FIGURE 12.1 A typical stationary anode X-ray tube.

The target is part of the anode assembly and is constructed of a material of high atomic number to achieve the best possible efficiency of X-ray production. However, even when the efficiency is as high as practicable, less than 1 per cent of the energy of the electrons appears as X-rays. The remainder appears as heat and so the target must have a high melting point and be able to dissipate the heat. This is achieved by constructing the anode of copper, which has a high thermal conductivity, with a tungsten target insert facing the cathode.

The copper anode is sometimes in solid form and has a finned radiator extending outside the tube to assist cooling. In higher power sets the anode is hollow and is cooled by circulating oil or water through it. In applications such as radiography it is important, in the interests of good definition, that the source of X-rays is very small. The filament is therefore mounted in a concave cup that focuses the electrons onto a small area of the target. Special measures are then necessary to prevent overheating of the target and the anode may consist of a rotating disc. The effective target area is then still small but the heated area is greatly increased and the tube may be heavily loaded without melting the target. This type of tube is used in medical X-ray sets, in which very high intensities and short exposure times are used to minimize difficulties caused by body movement.

12.2.3 Electrical supplies and controls

The electrical supplies required for the operation of an X-ray tube are a low-voltage supply to the filament and a very high voltage supply applied between anode and cathode. The supplies are usually derived from mains alternating current (a.c.). In the case of the filament supply, a step-down transformer is used to provide a voltage of about 12 V a.c. at a current which can be varied up to a few amperes. The tube voltage is provided by a high-voltage transformer which steps up the mains voltage (230 V a.c. in the UK) to the level required for operation of the tube. This is normally in the range from 5000 V up to some millions of volts, depending on the application. Since the voltage is derived from a.c. mains, the voltage between the anode and cathode is also alternating. A typical power supply is illustrated in Fig. 12.2.

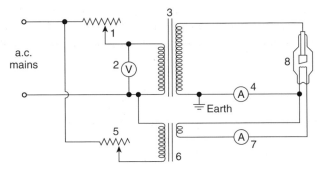

1. Tube voltage control   5. Filament current control
2. Voltmeter   6. Low-voltage transformer
3. High-voltage transformer   7. Filament current ammeter
4. Tube current ammeter   8. X-ray tube

FIGURE 12.2 Simplified power supply for X-ray set.

In a hot cathode X-ray tube electrons can flow only from the cathode to the anode since there is no source of electrons at the anode. However, the electrons will flow to the anode only when attracted by a positive voltage (remember that electrons are negatively charged) and so the tube will draw current and emit X-rays only when there is a positive voltage on the anode. The variation of the anode voltage with time is shown in Fig. 12.3. The shaded areas represent the periods when electrons are flowing to the anode (i.e. current is flowing) and producing X-rays at the target. The X-rays are not, therefore, produced continuously but as a series of pulses. If, for example, the a.c. supply is of frequency 50 cycles per second, then 50 pulses of X-rays are emitted per second. This pulsing is of some importance is designing X-ray monitoring equipment since a badly designed detection system could give a reading which depends on the frequency of X-ray pulses rather than on the

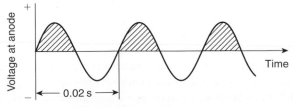

FIGURE 12.3 X-ray production in a self-rectifying tube.

average intensity. In some sets, special circuits are provided which smooth out the X-ray production to give a more uniform output with time.

12.3 QUALITY AND INTENSITY OF X-RAYS

The quality or energy of X-rays depends on the peak voltage applied to the anode of the tube. If the peak voltage in Fig. 12.3 is 200 000 V, this is expressed as 200 kV peak or 200 kVp. The maximum energy of the X-rays produced is 200 kV, but only a very small fraction will have this value and most of the X-rays will be of lower energy. The quality of the X-rays is, however, defined in terms of this peak energy and they are said to be 200 kVp X-rays. The penetrating power of X-rays is highly dependent on their energy. For example, the quality of X-rays used to radiograph a person's hand would be much too low to radiograph a 10-mm steel plate. The voltage on the tube is therefore set to give the appropriate quality of X-rays for each application. A few examples of suitable operating voltages and exposures for medical and industrial radiographic applications are given in Table 12.1.

Table 12.1 Typical operating voltages for radiography

		kVp	Distance (m)	Milliampere-seconds (mAs)
Medical diagnosis	Finger bone	40	1	10
	Skull	80	1	100
	Chest	80	2	80
	Pelvis	120	1	150
Industrial	6 mm steel	120	0.5	10
	25 mm steel	160	0.5	200

While the voltage on the tube controls the quality of the X-rays, the intensity is governed by the current flowing in the tube, that is, between the anode and cathode. This current, expressed in milliamperes (mA), is limited by the number of electrons ejected from the cathode. This is controlled by the temperature of the filament, which in turn depends on the current flowing in the low-voltage filament circuit. Since the dose rate is controlled by the tube current, the total dose in a particular case depends on the tube current multiplied by the time of exposure. The same dose would be received from an exposure of 10 mA for 1 s as for 1 mA for 10 s. In both cases the exposure is 10 milliampere-seconds or 10 mAs.

The dose rate from an X-ray set is very high compared with dose rates from typical sealed γ sources. The output is usually expressed in terms of the absorbed dose rate in mGy/min at 1 m from the set for a tube current of 1 mA. Some typical outputs are shown in Table 12.2.

The significance of the beryllium window mentioned in Table 12.2 is that at low voltages the penetrating power of X-rays is so low that a high proportion would be absorbed by a glass bulb. The use of a thin beryllium window minimizes this loss of output.

At higher voltages additional absorbers, or filters as they are known, are provided in the X-ray beam. It has been mentioned that X-rays of all energies up to the peak voltage are produced. Only the small fraction with the higher energies are useful, the remainder being undesirable in many cases. For example, in medical radiography, the low-energy fraction would not contribute to the radiograph, but would result in unnecessary skin dose to the

Table 12.2 Typical output of X-ray sets

Equipment and filtration	mGy/min/mA at 1 m
50 kVp beryllium window tube	100
100 kVp 3 mm Al (external to tube)	30
200 kVp 2 mm Cu + 1 mm Al (external to tube)	20
300 kVp 3 mm Cu + 1 mm Al (external to tube)	10
500 kVp 3 mm Cu + 1 mm Al (external to tube)	25

patient. The use of filters, usually an appropriate thickness of aluminium, selectively absorbs the low-energy or soft radiation without significantly affecting the useful beam.

12.4 PROTECTION AGAINST X-RAYS

12.4.1 General principles

Unlike radioisotopes, which emit radiation continuously, X-ray sets can be switched on or off at will. During operation the dose rate from the set may be very much higher than from small sealed sources. The equipment must be run in such a way that the operator does not expose any part of his body to the direct beam and no other person should be inadvertently exposed. The general principles applied to the protection of personnel are as follows:

1. Adequate training of all personnel who operate or use X-ray equipment in the correct operating procedures and in the hazards involved.
2. Limitation of the beam size to the minimum necessary by the provision of shielding and having collimators built into the set.
3. The use of suitable filtration to remove unwanted soft radiation.
4. Operation of X-ray equipment in a shielded room whenever possible. The controls should be situated outside the room and an interlock provided to prevent operation of the set while the door is open.
5. Provision of automatic visible and audible warnings that the set is operating or about to operate.
6. Confirmation of the effectiveness of the control measures by means of a system of personal and area monitoring.

The measures applied in any given case depend very much on the type of work and the local conditions. The main applications of X-rays are in industrial and medical radiography. This chapter deals with protection in industrial applications and research, and medical uses are considered in detail in Chapter 13.

12.4.2 Protection in industrial radiography

The main industrial application is in non-destructive testing of products, process plant and civil engineering structures. Testing of products is normally part of the production process and the testing is usually undertaken in purpose-designed enclosures with adequate shielding and appropriate safety systems to protect operating personnel. In other cases, radiography may need to be carried out in conditions that are far from ideal, such as on a construction site. In some applications, particularly where the size of the object requires more penetrating radiation, radiography is undertaken using sealed γ-ray sources, normally cobalt-60 or iridium-192.

The general principles that apply to the control of hazards from industrial radiography are as follows:

1. Non-destructive testing using ionizing radiation should only be used where it offers a clear advantage over other methods.
2. Whenever practicable, radiography or any other process using ionizing radiation from machines or sealed sources should be carried out within a shielded enclosure.
3. The control panel for the apparatus should be located outside the enclosure and devices should be provided to ensure that if any door of the enclosure is opened while the apparatus is energized, the apparatus is automatically de-energized.
4. For the protection of persons accidentally shut inside the enclosure, a means of communication is required to enable them to summon help. In addition, one or more of the following facilities should be provided for such persons:
   (a) means of exit:
   (b) means of de-energizing the apparatus; or
   (c) a shielded area.
5. Audible or visible signals (or both) should be given when the apparatus is about to be energized, and a different signal while the apparatus is energized. Where a γ-ray source is used, 'energized' means that the source is out of its shielded storage location and 'de-energized' means that it has been returned to its storage location.

Historically, the main problems have occurred when radiography is undertaken under site conditions, usually by contractors or subcontractors. Doses to radiographers have been quite high, and there have been cases of inadvertent exposure of other workers. There have also been incidents involving lost or broken sources. Recent changes in regulations have been aimed at ensuring that on-site radiography is only undertaken when it is impracticable to move the item into a proper shielded enclosure and that where on-site work does need to be undertaken it is properly planned and controlled. Before any radiography is performed under site conditions, a risk assessment needs to be undertaken to identify all the risks associated with the proposed work, including non-radiological risks. All reasonable measures need to be taken to protect others on the site, such as applying local shielding and physical restrictions on access. Consideration needs to be given to the possibility of accidents that could lead to increased radiation exposure and to measures to prevent such accidents or reduce their consequences.

12.4.3 Protection in research applications

The two main applications of X-rays in scientific research are X-ray crystallography and X-ray spectrometry. Crystals are regular arrangements of atoms and it has been found that definite patterns of scattered radiation, known as diffraction patterns, result from irradiating crystals with X-rays. The precise nature of the pattern provides important information on the structure of the crystals.

In crystallography, very high-intensity X-ray beams of small cross-section are used; these pose special health physics problems. In X-ray spectrometry substances are irradiated by X-rays and, as a result of absorbing energy, are excited and emit secondary X-rays. The energy of this secondary radiation is characteristic of the element producing it and so measurement of the secondary X-ray energies enables the substances to be analysed.

The precautions to be observed in this type of work include:

1. The apparatus should be adequately shielded and where access to the inside of the apparatus is necessary, either the machine must be automatically de-energized or effective steps must be taken to prevent the insertion of any part of the body into the beam.
2. Where a camera or slit-collimating system is in use the useful beam should be fully enclosed to provide adequate shielding.
3. Automatic visible or audible warning devices should operate whenever the apparatus is energized.

12.5 MONITORING OF RADIOGRAPHIC INSTALLATIONS

An important part of the commissioning procedure of any radiographic installation, or other facility which produces ionizing radiation, is a thorough radiation survey. Particular attention is paid to possible weaknesses in shielding, such as joints in the shielding material, viewing windows, doors and holes or ducts for services. The survey, which is usually performed at maximum tube voltage and current, is made under normal operating modes and then under other possible operating modes. Consider, for example, the case of a facility in which the X-ray beam is intended to operate in the horizontal plane and adjacent areas are shielded by thick walls. If the orientation of the set is changed and the beam operated in a vertical direction, would unacceptable levels of radiation occur in the areas above or below the facility? It should be borne in mind that if such a change is possible it is quite likely that, one day, it will be made. Even if the areas above or below the cell are unoccupied, high dose rates can occur outside shielding because of scattered radiation, often referred to as skyshine. If it is found that excessive radiation levels could possibly occur in adjacent areas, measures must be taken to prevent, or at least to give warning of, the situation. This can be done either by mechanically preventing the beam from being operated outside set limits, or by the provision of additional shielding or by the installation of area radiation monitoring equipment with warning signals. In general one of the first two methods is preferable.

Clearly, questions of this sort should be considered at the design stage but it is essential to confirm the safety of the facility by direct measurement. Surveys should be repeated periodically, particularly when any changes in operating procedure are introduced.

Care is necessary in the selection of instruments for monitoring X-rays. The major problem is that of energy response. Many instruments which are satisfactory for γ-rays and higher energy X-ray work seriously underestimate the dose rate from X-rays of below about 100 kVp. For low-energy work, instruments incorporating thin-window ionization chambers are probably the most suitable although they are sometimes lacking in sensitivity. Another possible problem when pulse-type instruments (e.g. Geiger–Müller tubes) are used is that the instrument may saturate in high X-ray dose rates and yet still appear to be working satisfactorily. This is due to the pulsed nature of the X-rays, which allows the instrument to recover between pulses. The instrument might then record the X-ray pulse rate rather than the average dose rate. This problem is fortunately rare in equipment of modern design but may arise as a result of a fault.

The safety of a facility is ultimately judged by the radiation doses received by operators and other persons working in the vicinity. These are normally measured by film badges, although many establishments now use thermoluminescent dosimeters. It is often worthwhile using a few film badges or other dosimeters to monitor fixed locations around the area on a routine basis. It should be borne in mind that personal monitors are small in area and X-ray beams, particularly in crystallography, may also be small in cross-section. It is quite possible for a beam to miss a personal monitor but nevertheless to irradiate the worker.

SUMMARY OF CHAPTER

X-rays: electromagnetic radiation; originate from changes in atomic electron energy levels or as bremsstrahlung when electrons strike high atomic number target material.

X-ray equipment: tube and a separate control unit.

    Tube: cathode and anode in evacuated glass tube.

    Control unit: high voltage supply controls the quality of the X-rays; the low-voltage supply to the filament defines the intensity.

Protection against X-rays: X-ray sets can be switched off but are hazardous when operating. Safety measures depend on the particular application but generally involve a combination of staff training, shielded rooms, filtration, warning systems, personal and area monitoring.

Site radiography: should only be carried out when it is impracticable to move item into a properly shielded enclosure. Full risk assessment, local shielding and physical restrictions on access are normally required.

Monitoring of radiographic installations: radiation surveys must be comprehensive and recognize the possibility of scattering into adjacent areas. Special problems associated with personal monitoring because of the small cross-sections of X-ray beams.

REVISION QUESTIONS

1. Describe, with the aid of a sketch, the operation of a hot cathode X-ray tube.
2. Compare the effect of varying the tube voltage and the tube current on the radiation output.
3. Compare the radiological hazards posed by large γ-sources and X-ray sets.
4. Design an enclosure for the routine X-radiographic examination of large metal castings. Indicate the safety features that are included.
5. What special problems arise in the monitoring of X-rays?

Radiation protection in medicine

13

13.1 APPLICATIONS

Ionizing radiation is a powerful tool in many branches of medicine, both as an aid to diagnosis and a means of therapy (treatment). For diagnostic purposes there are two basic approaches. The first is to pass a beam of radiation, normally of X-rays, through the body onto a detector such as a photographic film. The different degrees of absorption in the body produce a picture that gives information on the **structure** of the internal organs. For example conventional X-ray techniques can reveal broken bones, diseased lungs or the presence of a tumour. Another technique of great importance in medical diagnosis, based on the same principle, is **computed tomography (CT)**, popularly known as **scanning**. A tomograph is an image of a section, i.e. a slice, through an object, in this case the human body. The second diagnostic approach is to introduce a **radioactive tracer** into the body, for example by mouth or by injection into the bloodstream, and to observe its behaviour by means of external detectors. This technique can give information on the location and development of disease and **functioning** of body systems, such as cerebral blood flow.

The main therapeutic application of radiation is in the treatment of cancer. Radiation can induce cancer and yet, curiously, in some cases it can also cure the disease. This is because cells that are dividing rapidly are particularly sensitive to radiation and since cancers are groups of cells dividing in an uncontrolled manner, it follows that they are often more sensitive to radiation than normal cells. As with diagnosis, radiation therapy procedures can involve the use of beams of radiation to target the diseased tissue, or the use of radioactive materials injected into or applied to the body. Another technique, known as **brachytherapy**, involves the application of small sealed sources directly onto the site of the cancer. Clearly, the doses or levels of radioactive material involved in therapeutic procedures have to be very much higher than those used in diagnostic applications.

Those applications that involve the introduction of radioactive substances in liquid form into the body, whether for diagnosis or treatment, are generally referred to as **nuclear medicine** techniques. The dispensing, handling and application of the radioactive preparations, especially with the high levels of dose needed in therapeutic procedures, can give rise to radioactive contamination and so appropriate control procedures need to be applied. In particular, special measures are needed when dealing with patients to whom radioactive materials have been administered.

Techniques involving radiation and radioisotopes are of great value in medical diagnosis and treatment but it must always be borne in mind that the resulting radiation exposure involves risks that need to be weighed against the potential benefits. Until relatively recently, this was a matter for medical staff to decide and the general presumption was that the risks were trivial in comparison to the benefit to the patient. Under new regulatory regimes, however, all medical procedures involving radiation have to be shown to be justified and optimized to give maximum benefit to the patient.

13.2 GENERAL PRINCIPLES AND ORGANIZATION

Special problems arise in radiation protection in medicine because the well-being and reassurance of the patient is of prime importance. Also, a patient who has been given a large intake of radioactivity may represent a significant radiation hazard to others during their hospital stay. The normal methods of protection described in earlier chapters such as shielding, distance and containment cannot be applied in the usual way. However, with common sense, the patient can be adequately cared for without excessive risk to others.

The organization and responsibility for radiation protection in medical establishments vary from country to country. In the countries of the European Union (EU), national regulations are based on the general principles set out in Council Directives. In relation to protection of the patient, the relevant Council Directive is 97/43/Euratom of 30 June 1997. The important principles are summarized below.

1. Medical exposures should be justified by showing that they may be expected to produce a net benefit. This process of justification applies at two levels:
   (a) generic demonstration (normally at national level) that any new type of medical procedure is justified before it is introduced, and
   (b) the application of the procedure to an individual patient should be shown to be justified, taking into account the objectives of the exposure and the particular circumstances of the patient.
2. All medical exposures should be shown to be optimized. In particular:
   (a) in procedures undertaken for diagnostic purposes, the level of exposure should be as low as practicable, consistent with obtaining the required information, and
   (b) in the case of exposures for therapeutic purposes, the exposure should be individually planned and should ensure that the doses to regions outside the target volume are as low as reasonably achievable.
3. Optimization is also taken to mean that, in addition to careful planning, the best available techniques should be applied and that the whole process should be subject to quality assurance.
4. Procedures involving radiological exposure of patients should be undertaken in accordance with written protocols.
5. Clinical audits should be undertaken periodically to confirm the effectiveness of the procedures. These can be undertaken at the level of individual departments, medical establishments or at national level.
6. Responsibilities should be clearly defined. For example, in many cases, a medical professional (the referrer or prescriber) will refer a patient for a procedure to another medical specialist (the practitioner) who will decide on the details of the radiological procedure. A radiographer or a medical physics technologist (the operator) will then carry out the actual procedure, with support from medical physicists, particularly with respect to optimization.
7. All of those involved in the process should have adequate theoretical and practical training and should hold appropriate formal qualifications, diplomas, or certificates.

8. Special attention needs to be given to situations where there is a request for a radio-logical procedure involving a child, a pregnant woman or a breast-feeding mother. Special attention also has to be given to exposures where there is no direct benefit to the exposed individuals, such as volunteers taking part in research studies.
9. All radiological procedures should be performed in such a way as to minimize the dose to other persons.

The requirements for protection of workers in the medical field and of others who might be exposed as a result of medical procedures are essentially those that apply to any other industry and are set out in Council Directive 96/29 Euratom.

Each EU member state complies with the relevant Directives by means of its own internal legislation and regulations. In the UK, for example, all work with radiation is subject to the requirements of the Ionizing Radiation Regulations (1999), under the Health and Safety at Work Act (see Chapter 14). These apply to workers and to members of the public exposed as a result of the employer's activities. An additional set of regulations, the Ionising Radiation (Medical Exposure) Regulations (2000), applies to patients. Under both sets of regulations the ultimate responsibility for radiation protection lies with the 'employer'. In the case of hospitals under the jurisdiction of the National Health Service, the responsibility for the safety of patients, staff and members of the public rests with the Primary Care Trust. Their authority is usually exercised via a Radiological Safety Committee and a Radiation Protection Adviser (RPA). Since the RPA may cover many departments, or even several hospitals, it is usually necessary to appoint a Radiation Protection Supervisor (RPS) on a part-time basis in each department. In the case of patients, as set out above, responsibilities are separately defined for the referrer, the practitioner and the operator.

The key issues with regard to safety in medical situations are the initial and ongoing training of staff and the conduct of all radiological procedures within a strict quality assurance regime. This must ensure, among other things, that there is a clear chain of responsibility, that patients undergoing procedures are correctly identified, and that the procedure is appropriately optimized and conducted to give maximum benefit to the patient. It must also ensure that staff and others supporting or caring for the patient (such as family and friends) are adequately protected. It is emphasized that special consideration should be given before radiological procedures are applied to children or pregnant women. In the case of women who could be pregnant, the timing of procedures should take account of the last menstrual period. The application of nuclear medicine procedures, i.e. involving the administration of radionuclides, needs special attention if the patient is a breast-feeding woman.

13.3 DIAGNOSTIC PROCEDURES

13.3.1 Diagnostic radiography

Diagnostic tests involving radiological procedures are very common in modern medicine. For example, in the UK, some 40 million radiological examinations are performed each year. The great majority of these are conventional medical and dental X-rays but increasing numbers of more sophisticated tests, such as CT scans, are being undertaken. They may be carried out as part of the investigation of symptoms in an individual patient or as part of a general screening process. In the latter case, the tests are known a **asymptomatic** because they are not undertaken in response to reported symptoms but as part of a programme for early detection of certain medical conditions. An important example of this is mammography, which is made available to women in the 50- to 70-year age-group in order to detect early signs of breast cancer.

Until quite recently, most diagnostic radiographic tests were performed using X-ray sets in combination with photographic film. As a result of technological developments, these systems are gradually being replaced, at least in larger establishments, by direct digital radiography (DDR) systems. These use solid-state detection systems and have the advantage that the resulting image is stored in electronic format and can be accessed remotely by medical staff.

Whichever technique is used, careful selection of the X-ray quality (voltage) and the exposure enables good quality radiographs to be obtained with quite small doses to the patient. For example, using the best techniques available a chest X-ray can deliver as little as $100\,\mu Sv$ to the chest of the patient. With properly designed and operated systems, and with the minimum practicable beam size, the dose to other parts of the body will be much less than this. In some cases it may be necessary to take more than one radiograph, but clearly the number of 'shots' should be kept to the absolute minimum.

The dose to the radiographer is minimized by good design of the facility, for example, by the provision of a shielded cubicle in which the radiographer must stand to operate the set. Occasionally, difficulties arise; for example, young children may need to be held in the correct position. If a harness cannot be used it is better for the parent to hold the child rather than the radiographer, since the parent is unlikely to be exposed frequently in this way. A similar problem sometimes occurs in dental radiography when it is not possible to clamp the film in position in the mouth. In this case the patient should hold the film rather than the dentist or other members of the staff.

An important point to bear in mind in medical X-ray work is that a significant reduction in dose can be obtained with quite thin shielding because of the relatively low X-ray energy used (often less than $100\,kVp$). For example, lead-impregnated materials are available which can be made into aprons and gloves and are equivalent in shielding ability to approximately $1\,mm$ of lead.

In addition to the hazard from the primary beam, X-rays may be scattered from the patient or near-by materials, so constituting a further hazard. This needs to be considered when deciding how to protect the staff or members of the public who might be involved.

13.3.2 Diagnostic fluoroscopy

In fluoroscopy, the photographic plate used in radiography is replaced by a fluorescent screen. However, rather than the single short-duration pulse used in radiography, the X-ray tube remains on (or is continuously pulsed) during the examination. The screen fluoresces under irradiation and therefore gives a live picture. The principle of this technique is illustrated in Fig. 13.1, though it is emphasized that the arrangement shown is no longer used because of the high doses received by both the radiologist and the patient. Technology has moved on and the systems now in use are much more sophisticated. At currently acceptable levels of X-ray exposure, the image is faint and it is necessary to use an image intensifier to produce a picture that can be viewed by the physician. A further refinement is that the output from the image intensifier can be fed to a video system and this gives a record of the examination as well as allowing the medical staff viewing the image to be in a low dose rate area. In some types of examination, much higher quality images can be obtained, often with reduced dose, by injection of contrast media. These are chemical solutions that absorb X-rays more effectively than the body organs or fluids and so give enhanced images. This technique is commonly used in angiography, which is concerned with investigations of blood vessels.

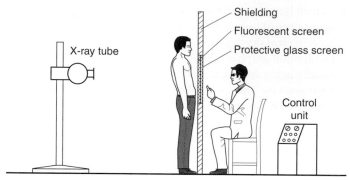

FIGURE 13.1 Principle of fluoroscopic examination.

Fluoroscopy is also used during interventional procedures so that, for example, a surgeon can view procedures being undertaken inside the body of the patient. A modern facility of this type is shown in Fig. 13.2. From a protection viewpoint, an important consideration is that the surgeon's hands may be within the X-ray beam for appreciable periods of time and the resulting doses need to be monitored and controlled. In addition, protection of the surgeon's eyes might be required because of back-scattered radiation, in which case either lead glass spectacles or a lead glass screen would be used.

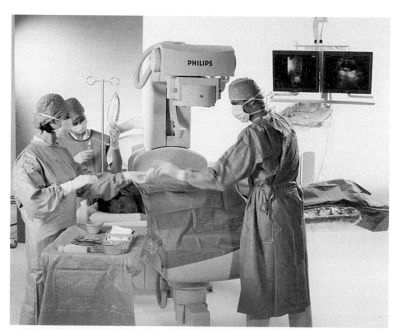

FIGURE 13.2 The use of fluoroscopy during surgery (Courtesy Philips Medical Systems).

In mass miniature chest radiography the patient stands in front of the screen in the usual way but the fluorescent screen is photographed using a small film. When a complete roll of film has been exposed the film is processed and the radiographs are viewed on a projection screen. The main advantages are economic since the costs of film, processing and storage are greatly reduced. The disadvantage is that the dose received by the patient is about 1 mSv or more compared with about 0.1 mSv for a conventional radiographic chest examination using best practice.

13.3.3 Computed tomography

Transmission computed tomography (usually shortened to CT) uses an X-ray tube and an array of detectors arranged in a supporting framework to rotate around the patient. A continuously rotating collimated X-ray beam passes through the body and the output from the detectors is analysed by a computer, which produces pictures of cross-sections or slices of the body. As in the case of fluoroscopy, the quality of the images can be greatly increased by injection of contrast media. The principle of operation is illustrated in Fig. 13.3, which shows a CT system in which the source and detector system are rotated around the patient as he or she is traversed through the system. A typical modern installation is shown in Fig. 13.4. Computed tomography is used for many types of radiological examination and is particularly useful for the diagnosis and follow-up of malignant tumours.

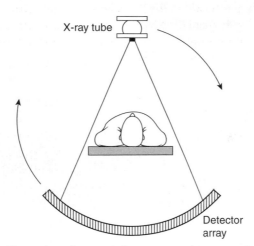

X-ray tube

Detector array

FIGURE 13.3 Schematic illustration of transmission computed tomography.

The dose received by the patient depends on the type and extent of the examination and would typically be between 1 mSv and 10 mSv, but only locally. The equipment is normally located in a shielded room with the radiographer located in an adjacent control room with a viewing window. In the event that the patient needs attention, the X-ray beam would automatically switch off when the door is opened.

Another similar diagnostic technique is **positron emission tomography** (PET), which involves injection of radioisotopes into the body. This is discussed later in this chapter under the general heading of nuclear medicine.

13.4 RADIOTHERAPY

It has been noted that the main application of radiotherapy is in the treatment of cancer. The aim is to deliver as high a dose as possible to the malignant tissue without causing excessive injury to surrounding healthy tissue. Typically, absorbed doses of a few tens of

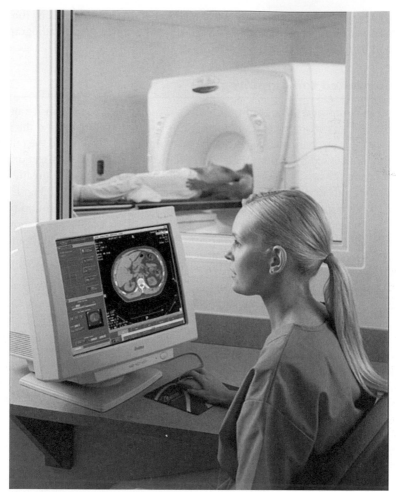

FIGURE 13.4 A modern computed tomography (CT) installation (courtesy Philips Medical Systems).

gray are required and they are usually delivered as a series of smaller doses, for example, 20 doses of 2 Gy at intervals of 2 or 3 days. This fractionation is necessary to reduce side-effects.

The most common method of treatment is by equipment such as linear accelerators able to deliver high energy electron beams of 6–20 MeV or high-energy X-rays of 6 MVp. Collimated beams of γ radiation from large Co-60 sources are also used. For treatment of superficial tissue, X-rays of about 200 kVp are often used.

In addition to selection of the appropriate energy, the dose to healthy tissue is minimized by varying the direction of the beam through the body. This is done either by using a different orientation for each treatment, or by continuously rotating the source around the tumour during the treatment. The principle is illustrated in Fig. 13.5 which shows treatment of a brain tumour using a rotating teletherapy unit containing a large cobalt-60 source. Although the tumour is being irradiated continuously, the surrounding regions are exposed for only a small fraction of the time. It is essential to use a well-defined beam and this is achieved by means of collimators.

Except in some low-voltage (<100 kVp) X-ray therapy, the problem of providing local shielding is such that the treatment must be performed in a shielded room with interlocks

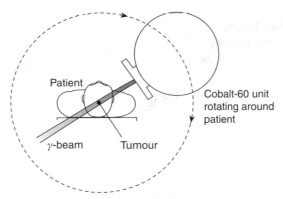

FIGURE 13.5 Treatment of brain tumour using cobalt-60 teletherapy unit.

arranged to shut down the equipment should the door be opened. A shielded viewing window and a means of communication with the patient are required.

All radiotherapy is carried out within an overall system of quality assurance. This requires a detailed treatment plan for the patient and the application of suitable quality controls at all stages. Usually, this involves a simulation system that includes a CT scan in order to define precisely the region to be irradiated. Often, a mould is produced for a patient and this serves both as a patient immobilizer and as a means of defining beam direction. The timing of exposures is under automatic control to ensure the correct dose to the target area. Regular testing and calibration of equipment (often daily) is a key aspect of quality assurance.

As noted earlier, radiotherapy can also be effected by brachytherapy which involves the application of small sealed sources into or adjacent to a tumour. The sources are normally applied either by surface applicators or inserted into body cavities or organs by specially designed delivery systems. In these cases, the exposure is fractionated, with individual exposures lasting from a few minutes to a few hours. In some cases, for example for treatment of prostate cancer, small radioactive seeds are surgically implanted and remain in the body delivering dose at a relatively low rate until the required dose has been delivered. The most common types of source used in brachytherapy are iridium-192, caesium-137 and iodine-125.

The source delivery systems are designed to minimize radiation exposure of staff. Where seeds are implanted into patients, special attention has to be given to the control of exposure of nursing and medical staff and controls need to be placed on visitors. Adequate protection can be achieved by sensible application of the principles of time, distance and shielding. In the case of sources that are re-used, regular leakage testing is required and written emergency procedures should specify the actions to be taken in the event of damage to or loss of a source.

It is possible, in some cases, for patients containing sources to be discharged. This is decided on a case-by-case basis, taking account of the radionuclide, the half-life, and the dose rate, which together define the risk to other persons.

Finally, it must be re-emphasized that whether using external beams of radiation, sealed sources or radioactivity injected into the body, the aim in radiotherapy is always to deliver a precisely predetermined dose to the target region while minimizing as far as possible the dose to adjacent healthy tissue.

13.5 NUCLEAR MEDICINE

The term nuclear medicine refers to the introduction of radionuclides in liquid (or occasionally gaseous) form into the body for either diagnostic or therapeutic purposes, or for the study of disease. Although the scale of application of these techniques is much less than for external radiation beam procedures, they are still commonly used practices. For example in the UK in the year 2000, some 700 000 nuclear medicine procedures were undertaken, of which about 98 per cent were for diagnostic and 2 per cent for therapeutic purposes.

In nuclear medicine, special attention should be given to women who are breast-feeding. Depending on the procedure involved, it may be necessary to advise the patient to cease breast-feeding until it is established that the risk to the child is sufficiently low. Precautions might also need to be taken to protect relatives, friends and others who come into contact with patients, particularly when they are discharged from hospital while still retaining radioactive material.

13.5.1 Diagnostic radioisotope tests

The purpose of radioisotope diagnostic tests is the investigation of body function. By introducing radioactive tracers in a suitable form into the body and observing their behaviour using external detectors, or by monitoring excretion, important information on the functioning of body organs may be obtained. The pattern of distribution of the radioactive tracer can be constructed by a γ-camera, which consists of an array of collimated detectors. Developments of this basic concept are now coming into common use, including **single photon emission computed tomography (SPECT)**. As the name implies, this is very similar to transmission CT except that the system detects γ-ray photons emitted by the radioactive tracers in the body and constructs an image of a section through an organ or the whole body. The organs that can be studied by this technique include the lungs, brain, liver, spleen, kidneys, thyroid, bone and blood. Most of these tests use suitable pharmaceuticals labelled with a radionuclide, commonly technetium-99m (Tc-99m). This has the great advantage that it can be obtained from a radionuclide generator. The generator typically contains 0.04 TBq of molybdenum-99 (^{99}Mo) which has a half-life of 66 h and decays to the pure γ-emitter Tc-99m which has a half-life of 6 h. The ^{99}Mo is absorbed onto tin dioxide and as the Tc-99m daughter is produced it is released into saline solution in the generator. The saline solution containing the Tc-99m is eluted into phials and, if necessary, combined with pharmaceuticals in preparation for administration.

Another technique used is PET. In this case, the radionuclide tracer is a positron emitter, usually fluorine-18 and the detection system detects the 0.51 MeV γ-rays from annihilation of the positron. These require greater shielding than the softer γ radiation from some other radionuclides. Less sophisticated, non-imaging, techniques are also used. For example for studies of thyroid function, the use of a single detector close to the thyroid yields information on thyroid function, see Fig. 13.6.

The quantities of radionuclides involved in these tests range from tens to hundreds of MBq and the dose to the patient is generally a few mSv. With increasing use of PET

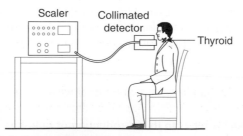

FIGURE 13.6 Thyroid radioiodine uptake test.

scanning, particularly involving the use of F-18, the dose received by staff involved in nuclear medicine procedures requires careful monitoring and control. With appropriate methods of working, fingertip and eye dose can usually be controlled and it is often the whole body dose that is limiting.

Under most circumstances the patient can be discharged immediately after the examination has been completed since the low activities involved do not represent a significant hazard to other people. The radioactivity is normally reduced to a very low level within a few days by radioactive decay and excretion.

13.5.3 Radioisotope therapy

In some circumstances radiation therapy is best performed by the ingestion or injection of radionuclide solutions into the body. Specific nuclides are chosen which concentrate in the organs requiring treatment, thus minimizing the dose to the rest of the body. The majority of therapeutic procedures involve the administration of nuclides of fairly short half-life (8 days or less) and the quantity is selected so that the required dose is delivered from the time of administration until the nuclide decays or is excreted. The main applications for radioisotope therapy are the treatment of thyroid cancer and thyrotoxicosis, using iodine-131. Typically, quantities of up to about 5000 MBq are administered for the treatment of thyroid cancer, giving a thyroid dose of up to 100 Gy, and a dose to the whole body of up to 1 Gy. Treatment for thyrotoxicosis, although more common than for thyroid cancer, involves only about one-tenth of the quantity of iodine-131 and therefore one-tenth of the dose.

Patients containing therapeutic quantities of radioactivity should be nursed under conditions that permit easy containment of radioactivity in case of contamination. Ideally, special rooms should be provided with en-suite facilities and all surfaces designed to permit easy cleaning. Where γ-emitters (such as iodine-131) are involved, the room may need to be shielded to ensure that the dose rate in adjacent areas is not significantly increased. The ventilation system should provide an adequate rate of air change, typically 5 10 air changes per hour, and should be designed to ensure that there is no possibility of the air being recycled to other areas. Protective gowns and gloves should be worn when handling the patient, contaminated linen or excreta and a special storage area should be provided for contaminated linen waste and samples of excreta. The RPS should specify any limitations on the time allowable for nursing procedures or visiting periods. Washing and monitoring facilities should be provided for use when leaving the area and regular radiation and contamination surveys should be made of the ward. Normally, liquid wastes and excreta are routed via a dedicated drainage system but discharge to the normal public sewage system where they are diluted by the much greater quantities of uncontaminated liquid from other areas.

In some cases, such as treatment for thyrotoxicosis, patients undergoing therapeutic nuclear medicine procedures may be treated as outpatients and discharged on the day of treatment. Where the administered quantity of radionuclide is higher, such as for the treatment of thyroid cancer, the patient would normally remain in hospital for a few days during which the level of retained radioactivity would rapidly reduce.

The source preparation is undertaken in conventional radiochemical laboratories and protection is achieved by the methods described in Chapter 8, that is, by minimizing the quantities of radioactivity handled, by containing it whenever possible and by the use of good procedures and facilities. The grade of the laboratory should be appropriate to the radiotoxicity and the quantity of the nuclides in use. It will be recalled that in such laboratories special attention is paid to surface finishes and to ventilation. Fumehoods are an essential feature even if quite low levels are being used. It is very important to have separate facilities for diagnostic and therapeutic work since low-level diagnostic tests can be ruined by cross-contamination from highly active equipment used in therapeutic work.

13.6 CONTROL AND DISPOSAL OF RADIOACTIVE MATERIALS

A large hospital may hold a large inventory of radioactive sources, both sealed and unsealed. One or more special storage areas may be required, located in positions that minimize the risk of fire or flood damage. The importance of keeping good records of the location of each source and the regular mustering of all sources cannot be over-emphasized. Leakage tests are required to be performed biennially on all sealed sources and any source showing significant leakage must be withdrawn from use immediately. Sources not in the main storage area should be kept and transported only in approved containers. These containers should be constructed to provide adequate shielding and adequate containment to prevent dispersal in the event of damage to the source. They should be clearly marked **radioactive** and carry the standard trefoil symbol. Written procedures should be available detailing the actions to be taken in the event of loss or breakage of a source.

Large sealed sources are subject to special requirements to ensure safe and secure retention and to avoid the possibility of accidents or misuse. Disposal of large sources is very costly and it must be ensured that sufficient funding will be available for this purpose at the end of their useful life.

In the UK, hospitals are required, under the Radioactive Substances Act 1993, to register their use of radioactive materials and to obtain an authorization to accumulate and dispose of radioactive waste. The general policy on radioactive waste disposal from hospitals is to use conventional local methods whenever possible. Solid wastes containing biological materials (known as clinical wastes) are normally collected in yellow plastic bags and sent for high-temperature incineration. The incinerator ash is disposed of, with other low-level solid waste, at a local refuse tip. As discussed earlier, low-level liquid wastes such as laboratory washings or excreta from patients are discharged to the normal sewage system.

Records must be kept of all waste discharges, both solid and liquid. It is not usually practicable to measure the activity and composition of the waste, but sensible estimates can be made from a knowledge of the quantities of the various nuclides in use.

The disposal of radioactive waste is described in greater detail in Chapter 11.

SUMMARY OF CHAPTER

Radiation is a powerful tool in medicine and is used in both diagnosis and treatment.
Justification: medical procedures involving radiation should be used only when there is a direct benefit to the patient.
Optimization: procedures should be optimized to produce the maximum benefit.
Diagnostic radiography involves the use of radiation beams, usually X-rays, to give information on the structure of internal organs. In most applications it uses photographic films but, increasingly, digital methods are being employed which means that the images can be stored on electronic media and accessed remotely.
Fluoroscopy is a means of obtaining moving images of physiological processes and so obtaining information on the functioning of body organs. The sensitivity of the procedure can in many cases be improved by the use of contrast media. Image intensification is

an essential part of the process if patient and staff doses are to be kept at an acceptable level. Great care is needed in the design and operation of a fluoroscopic facility to avoid excessive exposure of the patient and medical staff.

Computed tomography (CT): popularly known as scanning. Uses an X-ray beam and an array of detectors to build up a series of images of sections of the body. The quality of the images can be greatly increased by the use of contrast media. The equipment is normally located in a shielded room and the radiographer should not normally need to enter the room during a scan.

Radiotherapy: treatment by means of X-rays, γ-rays, electrons or neutrons; or small sealed sources. Beam therapy is carried out in a treatment room specially designed for the purpose. Close attention is needed in the design of shielding, interlocks and warning devices to minimize the doses to staff.

Brachytherapy: involves the application of small sealed sources directly onto the site of the cancer. Care is needed to prevent a patient containing a small sealed source becoming a radiation hazard to other patients and visitors. Areas where such patients are treated may need to be designated as controlled areas.

Nuclear medicine: the use of radioisotopes in diagnosis and therapy. This requires special attention to the design of laboratories and radioisotope departments for activities such as the preparation of radiopharmaceuticals and local storage, waste storage and disposal, radionuclide administration to patients, clinical measurements, sample measurements and decontamination. In diagnostic tests the nuclides used usually have short half-lives and low activity. In radioisotope therapy the procedures involve high levels of radioactivity and special precautions are necessary in the nursing of the patients in order to avoid the spread of contamination. Control needs to be exercised over nursing staff and those supporting the patient, such as family and friends.

Disposal of waste involves consideration of the permitted method(s) of disposal (e.g. to sewers and local refuse collection, subject to authorization), the quantities and activities involved, and the records to be kept.

REVISION QUESTIONS

1. What are the main applications of radioactive substances and other sources of ionizing radiation in medicine?
2. List some basic principles that are applied in the protection of patients and staff.
3. Discuss the various methods of diagnostic radiology that are available using sealed sources and compare their merits.
4. Describe the special radiological problems that may arise in the nursing of patients containing therapeutic quantities of radioactivity.

Legislation and regulations related to radiological protection   14

14.1 INTRODUCTION

The legislation and regulations dealing with radiological protection vary considerably from one country to another and are often intimately linked with other legislation, dealing, for example, with the control of nuclear energy. It is not possible to give an account of all the relevant national regulations in this book and readers who require further information on the regulatory position in a particular country should consult the bibliography. However, in most countries the starting point for the regulation of ionizing radiations is the recommendations of the International Commission on Radiological Protection (ICRP). The ICRP's recommendations are incorporated into wider international standards and guidance before eventually finding their way into national legislation. In this chapter the UK legislative position is considered in some detail and a brief account is given of the most important aspects of the regulatory positions in France, Germany, Japan and the USA.

14.2 RECOMMENDATIONS OF THE ICRP

The fact that the regulation of ionizing radiations around the world is remarkably consistent is due in large measure to the ICRP. The ICRP is a non-governmental scientific organization which has published recommendations about protection against ionizing radiations for over 70 years. Its authority is recognized world-wide and governments evaluate its recommendations and put them into practice in ways appropriate to their circumstances. The most recent recommendations of the ICRP were issued in 1991 in *Publication 60* (as discussed in Chapter 6) and most countries have now implemented them in their national legislation. Also, a group of six international organizations has prepared a set of basic safety standards for radiation protection, based on ICRP *Publication 60*. The group comprised the International Atomic Energy Agency (IAEA), the World Health Organization (WHO), the International Labour Organization (ILO), the Nuclear Energy Agency of the Organization for Economic Cooperation and Development (OECD-NEA), the Food and Agriculture Organization of the United Nations (FAO) and the Pan-American Health Organization.

Individual countries decide how to incorporate the recommendations of the ICRP, and any other internationally recommended safety standards for ionizing radiation, into their national regulatory framework. The UK, as a member of the European Union (EU), follows the procedures required of member states by the relevant treaties.

14.3 THE EURATOM DIRECTIVE

Members of the European Union are subject to the provisions of the Treaty establishing the European Atomic Energy Community (Euratom). A requirement of this treaty is that basic standards should be laid down in the Community for the protection of workers and the public against the dangers arising from ionizing radiations. These standards are promulgated via a Basic Safety Standards Directive, the contents of which must be given effect in the member states. The most recent Directive, adopted in 1996, takes account of the recommendations in ICRP *Publication 60*.

14.4 CONVERTING THE EC DIRECTIVE INTO UK LAW

In the UK most of the requirements of the Basic Safety Standards Directive are fulfilled by the Ionizing Radiations Regulations (1999) which came into effect on 1st January 2000 and which were drafted under the Health and Safety at Work (HSW) Act (1974). The HSW Act is a major piece of legislation which was enacted with the aim of rationalizing the existing, rather fragmentary legislation on the health and safety of persons at work, and of other persons who may be put at some risk by the activities of persons at work. The Act provided for the setting up of a Health and Safety Commission (HSC) which consists of representatives of employers' organizations, trades' unions and other organizations, such as local authorities. The HSC is responsible under the Act for formulating regulations, disseminating information to employers, employees and others, making arrangements for carrying out any necessary research and training, and generally providing advice on the interpretation of the Act. The Commission reports to the particular Secretary of State who is responsible for the activity or work area in question. The actual administration of the statutory requirements of the Act is the responsibility of the Health and Safety Executive (HSE) which comprises three persons appointed by the Commission. It is the duty of the Executive to make adequate arrangements for the enforcement of the relevant statutory provisions, except where such enforcement is transferred to some other authority (e.g. local authorities). The HSE enforces the various regulations through a number of Inspectorates which have been incorporated into the overall organization, e.g. the Factories Inspectorate, the Nuclear Installations Inspectorate, etc. The HSW Act is a very extensive and complicated piece of legislation and persons with responsibilities subject to the Act are advised to read the detailed regulations.

14.5 REGULATORY FRAMEWORK UNDER THE HEALTH AND SAFETY AT WORK ACT

The regulatory framework for radiological protection adopted by the HSC in 1999 consisted of a package which comprised the Ionizing Radiations Regulations (1999) and an approved code of practice entitled *Work with Ionizing Radiation*. This approved code, with its associated guidance, gives detailed advice on the scope and duties of the requirements imposed by the Ionizing Radiations Regulations (1999).

14.5.1 Regulations

The basic principle in the 1999 regulations is that all necessary steps should be taken to reduce so far as is reasonably practicable the extent to which people are exposed to ionizing radiation. This means that it is not sufficient merely to observe the dose limits specified in the regulations; there is a further requirement to weigh the costs of the possible health detriment from exposure against the costs of reducing or eliminating that exposure. In drawing up plans to restrict exposure, the regulations require the use of dose constraints, where appropriate. Dose constraints, as a tool to assist the process of optimization, were introduced in ICRP *Publication 60*. They are intended to be used solely in a prospective way to help ensure, at the design stage, that no new practice 'uses up' a disproportionate amount of the relevant dose limit. Although useful in theory, experience has shown that it is difficult to avoid confusing constraints with dose limits and investigation levels, and the ICRP is looking again at their usefulness.

Additionally, the regulations specify a dose value, set at three-quarters of the annual dose limits for workers aged 18 years or over. If this dose value is exceeded, an investigation must be carried out to ensure that doses are being kept as low as reasonably practicable and to initiate remedial measures if they are not.

The dose limits specified in the regulations for various categories of persons (workers, trainees, members of the public, women of reproductive capacity) refer to the sum of all radiation absorbed and committed from both external and internal sources, whether to the whole body or part of the body, arising from work activities. The basic dose limit specified in the regulations for the effective dose to any employee of 18 years or above is 20 mSv in any calendar year. However, where an employer is able to demonstrate that this dose limit is impracticable, an effective dose limit of 100 mSv in any period of five consecutive years may be used, subject to a maximum effective dose of 50 mSv in any single calendar year. In practice, UK employers have generally adopted the 20 mSv annual effective dose limit, with a lower limit (6 mSv) for trainees under 18 years of age. The limit on effective dose for any other person is set at 1 mSv in any calendar year.

The 1999 regulations also specify individual dose limits for the lens of the eye, the skin and the hands, forearms, feet and ankles. The limit on equivalent dose for the abdomen of a woman of reproductive capacity who is at work is 13 mSv in any consecutive period of 3 months.

To facilitate the control of doses, the regulations require controlled and supervised areas to be identified where persons need to follow special procedures to restrict exposure or where there is a likelihood of receiving equivalent doses in excess of three-tenths and one-tenth respectively of the annual dose limit for workers aged 18 years or over. Any person entering a controlled area must be designated a classified person unless he or she enters under a written system of work designed to ensure that no significant dose can be received.

Other regulations deal with appointed doctors and with the review of medical findings. There has to be a system for regular assessment of doses received by classified persons, and dosimetry services approved by the HSE must be used for this purpose. In addition, there are requirements to:

- provide appropriate safety devices, warning signals, handling tools, etc.;
- leak-test radioactive sources;
- provide protective equipment and clothing and test them;
- monitor radiation and contamination levels;
- store radioactive substances safely;

- design, construct and maintain buildings, fittings and equipment so as to minimize contamination; and
- make contingency arrangements for dealing with foreseeable but unintended incidents.

Where large quantities of radioactive substances are held there is a requirement to make a survey of potential hazards and prepare a report, a copy of which has to be sent to the HSE.

There are requirements for people to notify the HSE when they use ionizing radiation and to carry out a prior assessment of the risks arising from their work with ionizing radiations. The HSE must also be notified where there is a release or loss of radioactive substances, and when someone has received an excessive dose of radiation. Local investigations of excessive doses have to be made and records kept.

The provision of information on potential hazards and the instruction and training of people involved with ionizing radiation are required by the regulations. In addition, there are requirements to formulate written local rules covering all radiation protection arrangements and to provide supervision of work involving ionizing radiation; this normally necessitates the appointment of a radiation protection supervisor (RPS). Furthermore, the regulations require radiation protection advisers (RPAs) to be appointed whenever expert advice is needed and specifically whenever an employer has to designate one or more controlled areas.

As regards medical exposures, the doses received by patients undergoing diagnosis or treatment involving the use of ionizing radiation are not taken into account in determining compliance with dose limits. However, doses received by patients as a result of other patients' medical exposures are taken into account. In addition, there is a requirement generally to ensure that the clinical objectives of diagnosis or treatment are achieved with the minimum exposure.

14.5.2 Approved code of practice and other guidance

The Ionizing Radiations Regulations (1999) contain the fundamental requirements for control of exposure to ionizing radiation. Details of acceptable methods of meeting those requirements are given in the supporting Approved Code of Practice. An approved code of practice does not, in itself, have any legal standing but it would be taken into account by a court when deciding whether or not a person or organization had failed to comply with the regulations under the HSW Act. The code of practice is couched in much more understandable terms than the regulations governing it and it can explain the reason for the procedure which is included and thus aid the reader's understanding.

14.5.3 Prior risk assessment

Regulation 7 of the Ionizing Radiations Regulations (1999) requires that:

'before a radiation employer commences a new activity involving work with ionizing radiation in respect of which no risk assessment has been made by him, he shall make a suitable and sufficient assessment of the risk to any employee and other person for the purpose of identifying the measures he needs to take to restrict the exposure of that employee or other person to ionizing radiation.'

This means that, before any new radiation work commences, the responsible person, usually the work supervisor, must ensure that a risk assessment is made which identifies the hazards and evaluates the risks to both workers and any other persons who may be exposed. This risk assessment must be 'suitable and sufficient' and, to ensure this, the responsible person should adopt a systematic approach, which is almost invariably helped by some degree of quantification. However, it is important to realize that quantification cannot remove the inherent uncertainty associated with any risk and this needs to be recognized when formulating risk management strategies.

The basis of all risk assessments is to ask a series of 'what if?' questions (e.g. 'What if the containment should fail?') and ensure that the answers are as comprehensive and accurate as possible. The answers are obtained by reference to practical experience of similar situations, experts' judgement, manufacturing standards and test results, etc. The risk analyst then estimates the probabilities and consequences of all the foreseeable operating conditions that could arise, including non-standard operations, and makes an assessment of the overall risk. He then has to decide how to present the information so that it will be of maximum value in reaching decisions about the most appropriate control measures to be adopted.

Note that it is very important to adopt an approach that is appropriate to the degree of complexity and potential impact of each individual situation. For example, it would be unnecessary and inappropriate to apply the complex probabilistic risk assessment techniques used for evaluating the risks from nuclear reactors to the much more straightforward case of the risks to a glove box operator in a radiochemical laboratory.

Nevertheless, even for this relatively simple situation, if the risk assessment is to be considered suitable and sufficient, the following aspects should be given careful consideration:

- the nature and magnitude of the sources of ionizing radiation to be used, or likely to be present;
- the nature of the work to be carried out;
- the results of any previous personal dosimetry or area monitoring relevant to the proposed work;
- estimated radiation dose rates to which any person could be exposed as a result of the process;
- the likelihood of contamination arising and being spread;
- estimated levels of airborne and surface contamination;
- control of access to the working area;
- any control measures already in place;
- availability and effectiveness of personal protective equipment;
- possible accident situations, their likelihood and potential severity (spillages, failure of control measures such as interlocks, fume cupboards, ventilation systems, etc.).

When completed, a prior risk assessment such as this should provide the basis for making decisions about how to **manage the risk** and ensure that it is made as low as reasonably achievable (ALARA).

It is instructive to consider how risk is assessed by reference to the example of fluoroscopic examination illustrated in Fig. 13.1. In order to obtain the benefits of a 'real time' fluoroscope examination, giving a moving picture of the relevant part of the patient, the beam must remain on for a significant time, e.g. 30 s or more. For accurate diagnosis it is necessary to give the patient quite high dose rates, e.g. 10–20 mSv/min, but it would be quite unacceptable for the radiologist to receive such high dose rates, given that he/she is likely to be carrying out many such examinations each day. Therefore, the designers of the facility must ensure that the thickness of the screen and the amount of lead shielding incorporated around the screen are sufficient to reduce the dose rate to the operator to an acceptable level, provided that he or she remains behind the screen/shielding all the time that the X-ray beam is on. However, it is not sufficient for the designer to stop at this point. He/she must ask themselves how it might be possible for an operator to defeat these elementary precautions.

They should, for example, ask 'What if the operator has to move out from behind the screen to switch the beam on or off, or to adjust the patient's position?' 'What if the operator forgets to switch the beam off before moving out from behind the screen?' As far as possible these possibilities should be eliminated by the design of the system but, where this is not practicable, specific operating instructions and guidance should be produced to ensure that the exposures of both the operator and the patient are made ALARA.

See Chapter 13, Section 13.3.2, for an indication of some of the precautions that are frequently taken to minimize the risks during fluoroscopic examinations.

EXAMPLE 14.1

For the fluoroscopic examination procedure illustrated in Fig. 13.1, write down at least three 'What if?' questions that would help you to assess the possible accidental risks that might arise during the procedure. Explain, in qualitative terms, how you would go about assessing the magnitude of these risks.

14.6 OTHER RELEVANT UK LEGISLATION

There are several other pieces of UK legislation which have an impact on radiation protection (see Table 14.1).

Table 14.1 Summary of UK regulations

Regulation	Main provisions
Atomic Energy Act (1946)	Promotion and control of atomic energy development
Radioactive Substances Act (1948)	Control of radioactive substances and radiation apparatus
Radioactive Substances Act (1993)	Regulations on keeping and use of radioactive material and the disposal of radioactive waste
Nuclear Installations Act (1965, 1969)	Deals with licensing and insurance of specified sites which have substantial radiological hazards
Radiological Protection Act (1970)	Set up National Radiological Protection Board and Advisory Committee to provide various national services in the radiation protection field
Health and Safety at Work, etc., Act (1974)	Set up Health and Safety Commission and Health and Safety Executive to administer regulations concerning the health and safety of persons at work, and of other persons who may be put at risk by the activities of persons at work
The Ionizing Radiations Regulations (1999)	The regulatory package consists of the regulations and an approved code of practice plus more detailed guidance

14.7 BRIEF SUMMARY OF INTERNATIONAL GUIDANCE AND REGULATIONS IN OTHER COUNTRIES

In Section 14.3 the EU Directive on radiological protection was discussed. This Directive lays down the basic standards for the protection of workers and the public against the dangers arising from ionizing radiations within member states. It is binding on member states with regard to the results which have to be achieved. The Euratom treaty also requires member states to make appropriate provisions to ensure compliance with the basic standards and it also requires that provisions on radiological protection be communicated to the Commission to achieve the harmonization of such provisions in member states.

Other organizations which undertake work at international level to formulate radiation protection standards are:

The International Commission on Radiological Protection, ICRP (see Chapter 6).

The International Atomic Energy Agency, which produces 'Basic Standards for Radiation Protection', in collaboration with other international organizations (the governments of member states are invited to use these as a basis for formulating national legislation on radiation protection). In addition, IAEA has published a number of expert studies in the form of codes of practice, which give practical safety guidelines for specific applications.

The World Health Organization has published various reports concerning radiological protection and has collaborated with IAEA and other organizations in producing a number of guides on the protection of the public and workers against nuclear hazards. However, the WHO has not issued any regulations in this field.

The International Labour Organization adopted, in 1960, a convention concerning the protection of workers against ionizing radiations. In 1963 the ILO published a manual of industrial radiation protection which contains a model code of safety regulations concerning ionizing radiations, plus several guides for specific areas.

The Nuclear Energy Agency (NEA) of the OECD issues radiation protection norms from time to time. These norms are based on ICRP recommendations and are revised periodically to take account of the latest ICRP recommendations. In addition, NEA has sponsored or participated in the preparation of a number of studies in the field of radiological safety and collaborates with other international organizations in the establishment of safety standards.

The legislation and regulations dealing with radiological protection in individual countries are quite diverse and complicated, and it is beyond the scope of this book to attempt a discussion of them. Readers who wish to pursue this topic further should consult the bibliography. However, the regulatory frameworks in four major nuclear countries, France, Germany, Japan and the USA, are briefly outlined below.

14.7.1 France

As a member of the EU France complies with the requirements of the Directive through a number of decrees and ministerial circulars. The Ministers primarily concerned with radiological protection are:

- the Minister for Scientific and Industrial Development, responsible for atomic energy and whose jurisdiction includes the Commissariat a l'Energie Atomique;

- the Minister for Public Health and Social Security, who is responsible for safeguarding health and ensuring the health and welfare of the population. He controls the specialized technical department, the Central Service for Protection against Ionizing Radiations; and
- the Minister for the Environment, responsible for classified establishments.

14.7.2 Germany

Since it was not clear whether the Basic Law (*Grundgesetz*) covered all aspects of nuclear law, a special act supplementing the basic law was passed in 1959 for this purpose. Most activities relating to atomic energy are dealt with by federal legislation; legislative authority is left with the Länder (the German Federal States) only insofar as no federal legislation exists in the field. There is no single central body in Germany in which all the executive responsibilities concerning nuclear energy are vested. Supervisory and licensing powers are allocated either to the federal or land agencies as appropriate. The regulations dealing with the protection of the health and safety of the general public and of persons involved in work having radiation risks are laid down in the First Ordinance on the Protection Against Radiation Hazards and in the Second Ordinance on the Protection Against Hazards caused by Ionizing Radiations in Schools, both made under the Atomic Energy Act of 1959.

14.7.3 Japan

In Japan the control of nuclear energy is quite centralized. In general, the competent authorities responsible for licensing nuclear activities and for radiation protection are under the direct authority of the Prime Minister's Office. The Atomic Energy Act of 1955 laid down the main principles governing protection against radiation hazards. Under this act there is a further Prevention Law, which is aimed mainly at ensuring public safety by preventing radiation hazards that may arise from radioisotopes and apparatus generating ionizing radiation. Under the direct authority of the Prime Minister's Office are:

- the Atomic Energy Commission, which is in charge of preparing, examining and taking the necessary decisions on aspects such as the basic principles of protection against radiation hazards;
- the Science and Technology Agency (STA) which provides administrative support for the Atomic Energy Commission;
- the Radiation Council, a specialized body which establishes standards concerning radiation protection and levels of radioactivity.

14.7.4 United States of America

In the USA, the Nuclear Regulatory Commission has the prime responsibility for matters concerned with nuclear energy and the use of radioactive materials. The detailed requirements are set out in the Code of Federal Regulations, Title 10, Energy, known as 10CFR. Part 20 of 10CFR sets out the standards for protection against radiation, including permissible doses and levels of radioactivity in effluents.

Under the provisions of the National Environmental Policy Act of 1969, the Environmental Protection Agency has responsibilities in relation to the environmental impact of nuclear energy.

SUMMARY OF CHAPTER

ICRP: non-governmental scientific organization that publishes recommendations on protection against ionizing radiations. Most recent recommendations in ICRP *Publication 60* (1991).

Basic Safety Standards Directive: sets standards for radiation protection of workers and members of public which must be implemented in all EU member states. Most recent Directive adopted in 1996.

Ionizing Radiations Regulations (1999): converted most of the requirements of the Basic Safety Standards Directive into UK law. Supplemented by an Approved Code of Practice and other guidance.

Prior risk assessment: requirement of Ionizing Radiations Regulations (1999) that risk assessment must be carried out before any new radiation work commences. Must be suitable and sufficient.

REVISION QUESTIONS

1. Discuss the role of the ICRP in the regulation of ionizing radiations and explain why further steps are needed to incorporate ICRP's recommendations into national regulatory frameworks.
2. Discuss the relationship between the Basic Safety Standards Directive (1996) and the Ionizing Radiations Regulations (1999).
3. Explain what is meant by the term 'dose constraint'.
4. What are the dose limits specified in the Ionizing Radiations Regulations (1999) for workers and members of the public?
5. Give a qualitative outline of the steps necessary to produce a prior risk assessment for an active laboratory.

Health physics laboratory techniques

15.1 BASIC TECHNIQUES

In this chapter some of the basic techniques required in health physics laboratories are discussed. These include **radioassay**, which is the measurement of radioactive samples, and the calibration of health physics instruments.

15.2 RADIOASSAY

15.2.1 Identification of unknown samples

In general, the assessment of a radioactive sample, such as an air sample filter paper, requires not only measurement of the sample activity but also identification of the radionuclides present. Indeed, in most cases precise measurement of the sample activity is not possible without some knowledge of the nuclide and hence the type and energy of radiation emitted. The sample must, therefore, be analysed or else some assumptions must be made about its composition. It is not usually practicable or necessary to analyse every sample taken and so, in a particular area, occasional samples are analysed and the results are applied to other samples taken under similar conditions, perhaps with the introduction of a safety factor.

The characteristics of a nuclide which it may be possible to determine to enable its identification are the type and energy of radiation emitted, and the half-life. The methods by which these measurements may be made are described in the following sections.

15.2.2 Energy determination

The most convenient method of energy determination is γ-spectrometry, which was described in Chapter 7. For many commonly encountered radionuclides the observed spectrum enables rapid identification and measurement of sample activity. Similar techniques may be used for α- and β-emitters but the equipment is less readily available.

If the nuclide is a pure β-emitter or if the equipment available does not include a γ-spectrometer, reliance is often placed on β-absorption methods. These involve counting a sample in a β-counting system (e.g. a Geiger–Müller detector in a shielded castle) and observing the count rate with various thicknesses of aluminium placed between the sample and the detector. An absorption graph is obtained by plotting the count rate against the absorber thickness, usually on log-linear graph paper (Fig. 15.1).

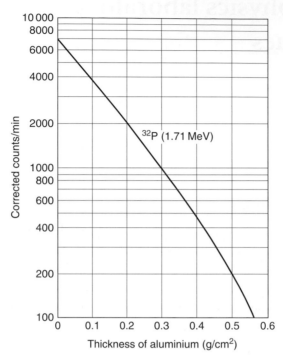

FIGURE 15.1 Typical β-absorption curve.

The basis of this method is that low-energy β radiation is more easily absorbed than high-energy radiation and so, by comparing the absorption curve with curves for β radiation of known energy, the β-energy of the sample may be estimated. The most precise method of determining the β-energy is Feather's method. This is described in detail in *Experimental Nucleonics* by B. Brown, to which the reader is referred.

A simpler but less precise method is to take a series of counts with increasing absorber thickness until the count rate has been reduced to about one-quarter of the initial value. The corrected count rate (see Sections 15.2.4 and 15.2.5) is then plotted against absorber thickness and the thickness that would reduce the count rate to one-half of the initial value is read off the bottom scale. This is the half-value thickness for that β-energy. An example of the method is illustrated in Fig. 15.2. The thickness of aluminium is expressed in units of grams per square centimetre (g/cm^2). This is obtained by multiplying the thickness of aluminium (cm) by the density (g/cm^3) to obtain g/cm^2.

The relationship between the β particle maximum energy and half-value thickness is shown in Fig. 15.3. Considering the sample in Fig. 15.2, the half-value thickness is $0.074\,g/cm^2$ and so, from Fig. 15.3, the β-energy is found to be about 1.4 MeV.

It should be mentioned that such determinations are not always easy because, in practice, samples often contain more than one nuclide and consequently several β-ray energies may be present. Even assuming that the β-energy is determined, this is probably insufficient to identify the radionuclide positively. A further indication may be obtained, in some cases, by measuring the half-life of the nuclide.

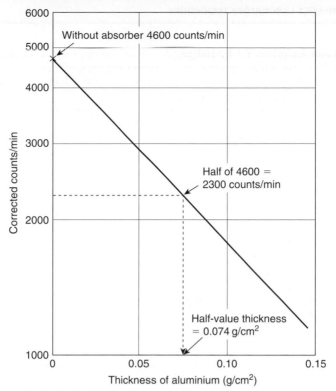

FIGURE 15.2 Determination of half-value thickness for β-emitter.

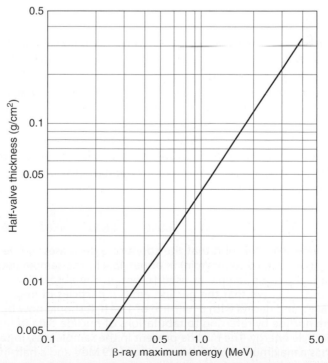

FIGURE 15.3 Relationship between half-value thickness and β-ray maximum energy.

15.2.3 Determination of half-life

The concept of half-life of a radionuclide was introduced in Chapter 2. It will be recalled that the activity of a sample at time t is given by:

$$A_t = A_0 e^{-\lambda t}$$

where

A_0 = the initial activity
λ = radioactive decay constant for the nuclide.

The half-life $T_{1/2}$ is the time at which A_t is one-half of the value of A_0, thus

$$\frac{A_t}{A_0} = 0.5 = e^{-\lambda T_{1/2}}$$

$$\therefore \log_e 0.5 = -\lambda T_{1/2}$$

$$-0.693 = -\lambda T_{1/2}$$

$$\therefore T_{1/2} = \frac{0.693}{\lambda} \text{ or } \lambda = \frac{0.693}{T_{1/2}}$$

It will be seen that the radioactive decay law can be written in an alternative form:

$$A_t = A_0 e^{-0.693 t / T_{1/2}}$$

In cases of nuclides having half-lives of between a few minutes and a few months, the half-life can be determined by taking a series of counts on the sample at suitable intervals (such that the count rate decreases by 10–15 per cent between counts). The corrected count rate is then plotted against time on log-linear graph paper, giving a straight line. The time to reduce the count rate to one-half of the initial value can then be read from the graph.

EXAMPLE 15.1

Using log-linear graph paper, plot a decay curve from the following data and estimate the half-life of the nuclide:

Time (h)	0	2	4	8	12	18
Count rate (counts/min)	6720	6050	5690	4563	3930	2989

It will be found from this plot that the count rate decreases to one-half of the initial value (i.e. to 3360 counts/min) in about 15.4 h. The sample used to obtain these data is the same sample as used to obtain the absorption curve in Fig. 15.2 and so it is known that the nuclide emits β particles of maximum energy about 1.4 MeV and decays with a half-life of 15.4 h. It should now be possible to identify the nuclide by referring to tabulations of nuclide data in order of half-life or β-particle energy. The nuclide present in the sample was, in fact, sodium-24 which has a maximum β-particle energy of 1.39 MeV and a half-life of 15.4 h.

As with β-absorption measurements, the procedure is often more difficult in practice because of the presence of more than one nuclide. This is illustrated in Fig. 15.4 which again shows a decay plot for sodium-24 but in this case a short-lived nuclide is also present. After an initial relatively rapid decay, the rate of decay decreases and eventually gives a straight line. The contribution from the longer-lived nuclide to the initial count rate can be obtained by extrapolating the straight line back to zero time. The half-life of this nuclide can then be obtained as before. To determine the half-life of the short-lived component it is necessary to subtract the extrapolated values of the count rate due to the long-lived nuclide from the observed count rate (i.e. the difference between the curve and the straight line is plotted). This procedure gives the decay plot for the short-lived nuclide and the half-life can then be determined. In Fig. 15.4 the short-lived nuclide is chlorine-38 which has a half-life of 37.3 min.

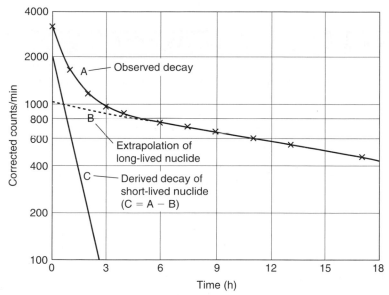

FIGURE 15.4 Decay curve of mixed ^{38}Cl and ^{24}Na sample.

15.2.4 Determination of sample activity

The conditions of measurement used in the radioassay of a particular radioactive sample depend on a variety of parameters, such as:

1. The activity of the sample.
2. The half-life of the sample.
3. The precision required.
4. The radiations emitted by the sample.

In general it is necessary to use a high-sensitivity counting system, comprising a radiation detector, a stabilized power supply, an amplifier, a discriminator and a scaler which registers the pulses received. (The basic features of counting systems are discussed in Chapter 7.) Often the detector has to be mounted in a lead castle to reduce the number of counts arising from the background γ radiation in the laboratory. The counts registered on the scaler must be corrected for background and may need to be corrected for the resolving time of the apparatus. It might also be necessary to calculate the appropriate statistical error.

In certain cases it is possible to mount a very thin radioactive sample at the centre of the sensitive volume of the detector and count all the particles or photons emitted; this is known as 4π geometry counting. In the more common counting systems only a fraction of the particles or photons emitted can enter the detector. The fraction of particles counted compared with the total number emitted is known as the efficiency of the counting system. The efficiency of a counting system is usually determined by placing a standard source in the appropriate counting position and determining the number of counts recorded in a fixed time. This is then divided by the emission rate of the source to obtain the counting efficiency. Usually, the efficiency is multiplied by 100 and expressed as a percentage.

EXAMPLE 15.2

A standard source of 220 Bq gives an uncorrected count of 2045 counts/min in a Geiger–Müller castle in which the background count is 65 counts/min. What is the efficiency of the system?

$$\text{Efficiency (\%)} = \frac{\text{corrected counts/min}}{\text{source emission rate, disintegrations/min}} \times 100$$

Corrected count rate = 2045 − 65 = 1980 counts/min. Now 220 Bq corresponds to 1.32×10^4 disintegrations per minute (dis/min). Therefore:

$$\text{Efficiency} = \frac{1980 \times 100}{1.32 \times 10^4} = 15\%$$

EXAMPLE 15.3

Calculate the activity of a source which gives an uncorrected count rate of 4925 counts/min in the equipment mentioned in the previous example. (Answer: 540 Bq)

Apart from the geometry of the counting system, a number of other factors influence the counting efficiency. These include backscatter, self-absorption in the source, absorption in the counter window and absorption in the air-gap between source and detector, all of which depend to some extent on the energy of the radiation. Ideally, the instrument should be calibrated with a source of the same nuclide and the same geometry as the samples to be counted. In the evaluation of routine samples for health physics purposes, a high degree of accuracy is not normally required and it is usual to calibrate the equipment with one typical source and to use the same calibration for the majority of samples. It is important to be aware that some nuclides, particularly low-energy β-emitters, can be seriously underestimated by this procedure.

15.2.5 Corrections for resolving time

When a charged particle or photon produces an interaction in the sensitive volume of a detector, there is a short period (usually of the order of 100 μs) during which further events cannot be recorded. This time is known as the resolving time of the apparatus and is the time required for the ions to be collected. It is sometimes referred to as the dead time of the detector because during this time it cannot respond to any new event. In many counting systems it is easier to introduce a fixed dead time into the system rather than determine the actual dead time experimentally. Since this artificial dead time is a function of known circuit parameters it has a precisely defined value.

Consider a circuit which has a dead time of 200 μs and suppose that it is used to count a sample which gives an observed counting rate of 500 counts/s. In recording 500 counts in 1 s the counter has been shut down for 200 μs after each count and was therefore inoperative for 500 × 200 μs ($=100\,000\,μs = 0.1\,s$). The 500 counts were therefore recorded in a counting time of only 0.9 s and so the true counting rate is

$$\frac{500}{0.9} = 555 \text{ counts/s}$$

This is written mathematically as

$$C = \frac{c}{1 - ct}$$

where

C = true count rate
c = observed count rate
t = dead time

Care should be taken with the units in this equation; if C and c are in counts/s, t must be in seconds (e.g. 200 μs = 200×10^{-6}s).

It is inadvisable for dead time corrections of much greater than 10 per cent to be applied, so when the counting rate is very high it is better to reduce it by changing the geometry.

EXAMPLE 15.4

Calculate the true counting rate of a sample if the observed counting rate is 15 000 counts/min and the dead time is 300 μs. (Answer: 16 216 counts/min)

15.2.6 Counting statistics

The radioactive decay of single atoms is random in time and so the number of particles or photons counted in a given time will fluctuate about an average value. The **standard deviation** (σ) is a measure of the scatter of a set of observations about their average value. In a counting system, if the average of a large number of counts is $\bar{N}$ then the standard deviation is found to be $\sqrt{N}$. Thus if:

$$\bar{N} = 400 \text{ counts}, \sigma = \sqrt{400} = 20$$

If a single count is made over a time t and N counts are recorded, the standard deviation on the count may be taken as $\sqrt{N}$. Usually, it is the counting rate which is of interest and this may be written

$$\text{counting rate} = \frac{N}{t} \pm \frac{\sqrt{N}}{t}$$

EXAMPLE 15.5

A 5-s count on a sample gives a result of 100 counts. What is the counting rate and the standard deviation?

$$\text{Counting rate} = \frac{100}{5} \pm \frac{\sqrt{100}}{5}$$

$$= 20 \pm 2 \text{ counts/s}$$

The significance of standard deviation is that 68 per cent of observations are within one standard deviation of the true counting rate. Hence, in the above example, there is a 68 per cent chance that the counting rate lies between 18 counts/s and 22 counts/s. The standard deviation is, therefore, a measure of the accuracy of an observation. In counting, greater accuracy can be achieved only by increasing the total count recorded. Thus, if in the previous example 1000 counts had been recorded in 50 s,

$$\text{counting rate} = \frac{1000}{50} \pm \frac{\sqrt{1000}}{50}$$

$$= 20 \pm \frac{31.6}{50}$$

$$= 20 \pm 0.63 \text{ counts/s}$$

or if 10 000 counts were recorded in 500 s

$$\text{counting rate} = \frac{10\,000}{500} \pm \frac{\sqrt{10\,000}}{500}$$

$$= 20 \pm \frac{100}{500}$$

$$= 20 \pm 0.2 \text{ counts/s}$$

Although the counting rate is the same in all three cases, the accuracy has been improved by counting for longer periods.

Standard deviation can also be expressed as a percentage, for example on counts of 100, 1000 and 10 000:

$$N = 100, \quad \sigma = 10 = 10\%$$

$$N = 1000, \quad \sigma = 31.6 = 3.16\%$$

$$N = 10\,000, \sigma = 100 = 1\%$$

For a count (or a count rate) to be accurate to 1 per cent standard deviation, the counting period must be long enough to give at least 10 000 counts.

Usually, we need to find the counting rate S resulting from a source superimposed on a background counting rate. If N counts are recorded in time t_1, due to source and background, and B counts are recorded in time t_2 due to background alone, then the corrected counting rate S is given by:

$$S = \frac{N}{t_1} - \frac{B}{t_2} \pm \sigma_s$$

where

$$\sigma_s = \sqrt{(\sigma_1^2 + \sigma_2^2)}$$

$$= \sqrt{\left(\frac{N}{t_1^2} + \frac{B}{t_2^2} \right)}$$

The general expression for this type of measurement becomes:

$$S = \frac{N}{t_1} - \frac{B}{t_2} \pm \sqrt{\left(\frac{N}{t_1^2} + \frac{B}{t_2^2} \right)}$$

EXAMPLE 15.6

A source is counted in a Geiger–Müller castle and registers 6720 counts in 4 min. The background is then counted for 10 min and gives 480 counts. What is the corrected count rate and the standard deviation?

$$S = \frac{6720}{4} - \frac{480}{10} \pm \sqrt{\left(\frac{6720}{16} + \frac{480}{100} \right)}$$

$$= 1680 - 48 \pm \sqrt{(420 + 4.8)}$$

$$= 1632 \pm \sqrt{424.8}$$

$$= 1632 \pm 20.6 \text{ counts/min}$$

When counting very low activity sources, very long counting times may be required to achieve an acceptable statistical accuracy. Under such circumstances it is desirable to choose the most efficient distribution of the time between the (source + background) and the background count alone. The highest accuracy is achieved when:

$$\frac{t_1}{t_2} = \sqrt{k}$$

where t_1 is time spent counting (source + background), t_2 is time spent counting background alone, and k is the ratio of total counting rate of (source + background) to the background rate alone.

It is often worthwhile, when confronted with a sample of unknown activity, to do a preliminary investigation of the counting rates to be expected. This entails a short (source + background) count, followed by a background only count, each count being for 1 or 2 min duration only. From these results the expected counting rates are determined roughly, and the length and distribution of time for the accurate assessment of the sample are calculated.

EXAMPLE 15.7

If the total counting rate for source + background is 360 counts/min and the background counting rate is 40 counts/min, what proportion of the total available time should be spent on counting background? (Answer: 25 per cent)

15.3 CALIBRATION OF RADIATION MONITORS

15.3.1 General

The manufacturer of an instrument is normally responsible for carrying out a detailed calibration procedure before handing it over to the user. The following items are normally investigated:

1. Sensitivity of the instrument under normal working conditions.
2. Energy response.
3. Rate response.
4. Temperature variations.

The importance of checking the energy response over a wide range of energies (usually 100 keV to several MeV) has been mentioned in Chapter 8. Similarly, if the instrument has several scales, as in most dose-rate meters, it must respond satisfactorily on all the scales. Temperature response should not be an important factor with laboratory instruments since it is always possible to select components that are practically unaffected by temperature variations.

The user of an instrument merely needs to know that the instrument is within specification when supplied and will subsequently carry out less extensive tests to check on its performance. Most instruments have built-in checks such as battery checks, zero adjustments and sensitivity checks. Generally, the user need only check the sensitivity periodically since this is the parameter that is most likely to change over a period of time.

There are basically two methods available for carrying out such checks:

1. Direct calibration using known standard sources.
2. Intercalibration with a specially calibrated instrument.

In the UK, all instruments have to be tested at intervals not exceeding 14 months and the results recorded in a special register. Similar requirements apply in other countries.

15.3.2 Direct calibration

When only a few instruments have to be calibrated it is usually sufficient to use a simple jig, as shown in Fig. 15.5. This jig ensures that the instrument and source are always positioned in such a way that constant geometry is maintained. Conversely, when many instruments have to be calibrated it is often necessary to set up a special calibration facility with free-air conditions (that is, minimum scattering around the source) and an accurately known source. One such facility is illustrated in Fig. 15.6. The instrument being calibrated is moved along a guiding track and positioned remotely. Readings are obtained via a mirror system.

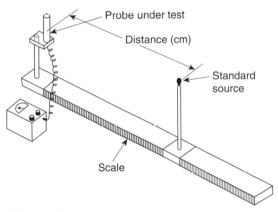

FIGURE 15.5 Simple calibration jig.

15.3.3 Intercalibration with specially calibrated instrument

When a calibrated instrument is available it is not necessary to have free-air facilities. All that is required is a system that will allow the radiation intensity to be varied over the range required. Such a system is shown in Fig. 15.7, where the radiation intensity is varied by altering the position of the source. The dose rate is measured using the specially calibrated instrument and then compared with the reading from the instrument under test. It is important to remember that, since no attempts are made to avoid scattered radiation in this test set-up, a variable proportion of the radiation reaching the detector will be degraded in energy. This does not matter when the standard instrument and the one under test have the same energy response. However, if their energy responses are different the results may be invalid.

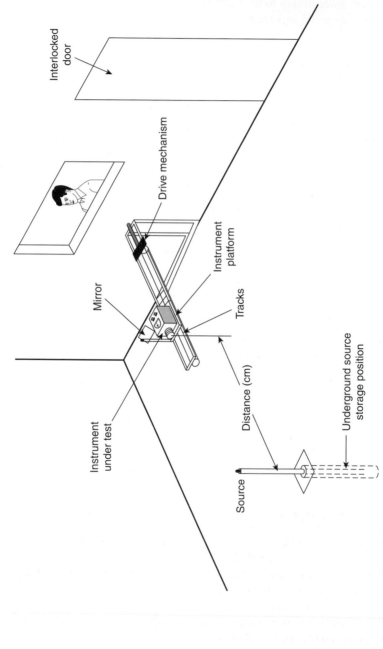

FIGURE 15.6 Shielded calibration room with remote operation (after Barnes and Taylor).

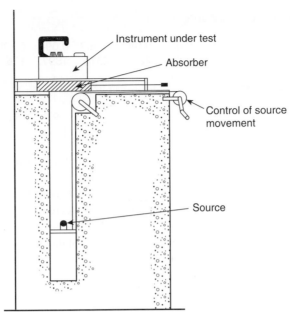

FIGURE 15.7 Layout for calibration using a standard instrument (after Barnes and Taylor).

SUMMARY OF CHAPTER

Radioassay: measurement of radioactive samples.

Identification of nuclides: α-, β- or γ-spectrometry, β-absorption or half-life measurements.

Determination of sample activity: counting efficiency, dependence on energy. Correction for counter background.

Resolving time: detector is inoperative for short time after registering a pulse; this reduces effective counting time and is important at high count rates.

Counting statistics: standard deviation (σ); a measure of the accuracy of a count. $\sigma = \sqrt{N}$. To achieve good accuracy counts must be large; 10 000 counts gives 1 per cent accuracy. Background count has an effect on accuracy.

Calibration of instruments: use standard source or compare with calibrated instrument.

REVISION QUESTIONS

1. Why is it usually necessary to determine the composition of the activity on an air sample filter paper? How can the nuclides be identified?
2. A sample gives a count of 16 347 in 1 min when counted in a Geiger–Müller counter of background 750 counts in 10 min, dead time 300 μs and efficiency of 15 per cent. Calculate the sample activity.
3. What is meant by the resolving time of a detector and what is its importance in counting measurements?
4. The results of β-absorption and decay measurements on a sample are shown below. Estimate the half-life and the maximum β-energy. Refer to nuclide data and attempt to identify the nuclide present in the sample.

Beta-absorption measurements

Absorber (g/cm²)	0	0.017	0.041	0.067	0.094	0.120	0.143	0.168
Corrected counts/min	3613	3324	2867	2310	1897	1563	1306	1097

Decay measurements

Time (days)	0	1	3	6	9	12	15	18
Corrected counts/min	3613	3376	3136	2637	2353	1980	1768	1510

5. What is the significance of the standard deviation of a measurement and how is its value calculated for a single counting measurement?

6. A sample is counted in a β-castle and registers 22 501 counts in 50 min. The background count gives 2040 in 30 min. Calculate the corrected count rate and the standard deviation.

7. It is required to calibrate a γ dose-rate meter using a standard source which is known to give 720 μSv/h at 1 m. The instrument is to be checked at dose rates of 200, 500, 1000, and 2000 μSv/h. Calculate the distance from the source to the instrument in each case.

Radiological emergencies

16

16.1 INTRODUCTION

A radiological emergency may be defined as any situation that gives rise to an abnormal or unexpected radiation hazard. This definition covers anything from a minor laboratory spill involving a few megabecquerels of radioactive solution up to a major reactor accident in which many thousands of terabecquerels of fission products may be released.

An emergency can arise because of:

1. A **loss of shielding**, resulting in high radiation levels.
2. A **loss of containment**, resulting in a release of activity.
3. An **uncontrolled criticality**, which is, effectively, the rapid generation of a large radioactive source and high levels of radiation.

Usually, these situations result from some conventional cause such as a mechanical failure, fire, flooding or a transport accident.

For planning and control purposes it is usual to differentiate between the various levels of emergency that can occur. The minor laboratory spills mentioned above are more of a nuisance than a danger and it is more appropriate to refer to them as **local incidents**. A more serious situation, perhaps requiring evacuation of certain areas, but having no effect outside the site or establishment is often called a **site emergency**. If the incident could be hazardous to the general population outside the site it is sometimes termed a **public emergency**.

In any event it is of great value to have analysed the possible occurrences in advance and to have formulated procedures for dealing with them. It is vitally important to detect any abnormal situation as quickly as possible. For example, if a loss of shielding accident is detected immediately and the appropriate corrective actions or evacuation measures taken, the dose received may be very small. Conversely, very large doses may be received if operating personnel and others in the vicinity of the plant are not aware of the situation.

In this chapter a number of situations of the types listed above will be considered.

16.2 LOSS OF SHIELDING

16.2.1 Small sealed sources

Small sealed sources, usually γ-emitters, are widely used in industry, medicine and teaching. It is unlikely that any source with an activity less than 100 MBq could result in an excessive dose to a person (unless, for example, it was carried in the pocket) and so the loss of shielding for such sources would probably be a local incident. Such sources are usually handled by tongs and stored in small lead-lined pots. The most common loss of shielding incidents occur when a source is removed from its container by some person who fails to return it. The best method of protecting against such incidents is to use installed alarm instruments which show when the source is out of its pot. Regular source musters minimize the possibility that the situation remains undetected for a long period of time.

The loss of shielding could also result from mechanical damage, for example, if the container were dropped, in which case there should be no problem in detecting the event. The possible effects of fires, which might not only cause the shielding to melt but also cause a loss of containment of the source material itself, must also be considered.

16.2.2 Large sealed sources

Large sealed sources such as those used for industrial processing or radiography and medical radiotherapy are usually housed in specially constructed containers with mechanical means for controlling the time of exposure. The containers are designed to withstand foreseeable mechanical accidents and to resist fire. The possibility of inadvertent exposure of the source is minimized by the design of the equipment, but alarm systems are desirable to detect any fault conditions.

The majority of accidents involving sources of this type have been in industrial radiography. This is often performed in difficult conditions on construction sites without any form of installed monitoring equipment. In a number of accidents the radioactive source became detached from the operating mechanism and when the mechanism was retracted into the storage position the source remained unshielded. In some cases the source was found by a person who placed it in their pocket without being aware of its hazardous properties. This resulted in very large, and sometimes fatal, doses being received. The prevention of such accidents depends not only on the correct use of appropriate equipment but also on good training and strict adherence to preplanned monitoring procedures by the radiographer. Various portable alarm devices are also available which can be used in field conditions.

16.2.3 Reactor fuel handling accidents

The problems and dangers involved in handling the intensely radioactive fuel from a nuclear reactor are described in Chapter 10. For large power generating reactors complex, remotely controlled handling equipment removes fuel from the reactor and transfers it to a cooling pond. It is virtually impossible, because of built-in safety devices, for fuel to become unshielded at this stage. With research reactors there is usually more scope for fuel handling accidents and greater reliance has to be placed on following approved operating procedures. There is greater scope for loss of shielding accidents in fuel cooling ponds, perhaps through the inadvertent withdrawal of fuel from the pond or because of loss of water. The possibility of such occurrences is minimized by good equipment design and careful operation and maintenance but, as a final safeguard, an installed radiation alarm system is essential.

16.3 LOSS OF CONTAINMENT

16.3.1 Minor spillage of radioactivity

Perhaps the most common 'abnormal occurrence' in a laboratory is a minor spillage of up to a few megabecquerels of radioactive solution. The frequency of such events is minimized by good laboratory practices such as keeping containers of radioactive solutions in trays to contain any spillage. Spills do, however, occur even in the best regulated laboratories but if they are dealt with correctly, the contamination and therefore the incident should not spread outside the laboratory or area in which it occurred. After carrying out any personnel decontamination that may be required, the most important action is to clean up the activity using absorbent materials before it dries out and becomes airborne.

A useful precaution in laboratories handling unsealed sources is to have available a few **spillpacks**. A spillpack is simply a plastic bag containing a pair of gloves, a pair of overshoes and a wad of absorbent material (cotton waste, paper towels, etc.). When a spill occurs, the gloves and overshoes are donned and the spill is wiped up using the absorbent material which is then replaced in the bag for disposal. Having quickly cleaned up the bulk of the activity the surface can then be monitored and decontaminated further if necessary. If any person is contaminated as a result of the spill, they should put on the clean gloves and overshoes and go to a change or decontamination area without spreading contamination.

Any spillage that remains undetected for some time is likely to cause problems because it will be spread around, and possibly outside, the area. This is why it is important for people working in areas in which unsealed sources are used to make a habit of washing and monitoring each time they leave the area.

A release of activity can also result from a failure of services such as ventilation or electrical supplies. Glove boxes can pose a particular problem in this respect. A glove box is normally operated at a pressure slightly below atmospheric, which means that leakage tends to be in, rather than out. If some failure causes the box to pressurize, outward leakage may occur or, more seriously, a glove or panel may be blown out resulting in a minor release. Specific attention needs to be paid in the design to such possibilities in order to minimize the chances of them occurring and there should be preplanned procedures for dealing with them.

16.3.2 Major spills of radioactivity

A major spill, involving 100 MBq or so of activity, could result in a serious incident, the seriousness of which will depend on the radiotoxicity of the nuclides involved. Immediate evacuation of personnel might be required together with shutdown of the ventilation system and sealing the area off to contain the spread of activity. A controlled re-entry to the area by a team wearing appropriate protective clothing and respirators might be necessary. It is circumstances such as these that demonstrate the value of a properly designed laboratory. Decontamination is a relatively simple matter in a good laboratory where proper attention has been paid to surface finishes. In badly designed laboratories, decontamination may be difficult or even impossible.

16.3.3 Major releases from nuclear facilities

Potentially the most serious loss of containment accidents involve the release of fission products from a reactor. It will be recalled that the fission products are contained within three separate boundaries: the fuel cladding, the boundary of the cooling system and the reactor building. In a power reactor, the most likely cause of a fission product release is a failure of the pressure circuit (e.g. a fracture of a coolant duct) resulting in a loss of coolant, with subsequent overheating and meltdown of the fuel. Fission products would then be released from the molten fuel and escape through the breach in the cooling system. In a large reactor, if only 0.1 per cent of the fission product inventory leaked from the cooling system this could amount to over 10^{17} Bq. If 1 per cent of this amount then escaped from the reactor building or containment, the release to the environment would be 10^{15} Bq. This would result in very high levels of radiation and contamination on the reactor site. It would also be a hazard to the local population and hence a public emergency.

It was considerations such as this that led to the siting of the first generation of nuclear reactors in remote areas. Some large plants of more recent design have been sited quite close to towns. This is justified either because, in plants such as the advanced gas-cooled reactor (AGR), the entire reactor system is inside a massive prestressed concrete pressure vessel and a failure of this is virtually inconceivable, or because other reactor systems such as light water reactors (LWR) have special systems, including containment structures, to minimize the release of radioactivity in the event of a failure of the coolant system.

One of the earliest reactor accidents occurred at Windscale, Cumbria, UK, in 1957. The reactor was of a very early design and used direct-cycle air cooling, i.e. air was drawn in through the reactor core, removing heat, and was discharged back to the atmosphere through filters and a tall stack. A special operation was being performed which caused the fuel rods to overheat and catch fire. The main activity released was iodine-131 which, being a vapour, was not removed very effectively by the filters. An estimated 7×10^{14} Bq of iodine-131 was released and, although evacuation of the local population was not necessary, milk produced in a large area downwind of the site was declared unfit for consumption. This was because of the exposure pathway:

$$\text{Iodine-131} \longrightarrow \text{pasture} \longrightarrow \text{uptake by cows} \longrightarrow \text{milk}$$
$$\text{consumption of milk} \longrightarrow \text{dose to thyroid.}$$

Other fission products such as strontium and caesium were also released but, because of the absorptive action of the filters, in much smaller quantities.

Direct-cycle air cooling is no longer used on power reactors and so further accidents of this type are not possible. A great deal was learned from the Windscale accident about the sort of organization, equipment and procedures that are necessary to deal with major accidents.

In 1979, an accident occurred at a large commercial pressurized water reactor (PWR) plant at Three Mile Island (TMI), Pennsylvania, USA. The accident followed a major leak in the pressure system and the failure of a safety system to operate because of an incorrectly aligned valve. The resulting loss of cooling led to overheating of fuel and release of activity to the environment via the gas waste system. The released activity consisted mainly of short-lived inert fission product gases, so the resulting radiation exposure of the surrounding population was low. However, some evacuation was undertaken, mainly of young children and pregnant women, and the accident had a considerable adverse effect on public attitudes to nuclear power in the USA.

The TMI accident led to increased efforts to understand the processes that would occur during a severe reactor accident. It now seems that, for the majority of accidents that might occur on LWRs, the release of fission products would be considerably less than had previously been thought. This is because various processes within the containment, and the containment structure itself, are very effective in limiting the release.

A much more serious reactor accident occurred at Chernobyl, Ukraine, in 1986 and involved a 1000 MWe (megawatt electrical) graphite moderated boiling water reactor, a design peculiar to Eastern Europe. The accident resulted in a major fire and a large release of radioactivity (about 1000 times the amount released in the Windscale accident and a million times the amount released at TMI). Extremely high on-site dose rates occurred and there was extensive contamination, not just in the vicinity of the site but across wide areas of Western Europe. The town of Pripyat (3–5 km from the site), with a population of 45 000, was evacuated in under 3 h on the afternoon of the second day of the release. At that time, dose rates in the part of Pripyat closest to the site were in the range 7–10 mSv/h. It has been estimated that the majority of Pripyat's inhabitants received whole body γ doses of 15–50 mGy and 100–200 mGy β skin doses.

Nearly two decades later, the Chernobyl accident continues to dominate world-wide thinking about the radiological consequences of nuclear reactor accidents. Epidemiological studies of the effects of the release on the various affected populations continue to determine treatment regimens, particularly for thyroid cancers in children, and to refine the risk factors. The accident has led to a complete reappraisal of the methods for modelling the release, transport and uptake of radionuclides, and of the preparations and procedures that are needed to handle such situations. In particular, it has resulted in an International Convention on Nuclear Safety which is intended to improve the safety of all nuclear plants world-wide and a Convention on Early Notification of a Nuclear Accident to ensure that all potentially affected countries are notified rapidly of any future nuclear incident.

Other potential sources of a major release of radioactivity are nuclear fuel reprocessing plants and the waste storage facilities associated with them. As explained in Chapter 10, after the fuel has been chemically processed the highly active waste stream, which contains almost all the fission products and higher actinides, is routed into special storage tanks. These tanks may contain several cores' worth of activity and have to be cooled to remove the radioactive decay heat and prevent the build-up of potentially explosive hydrogen gas. Any sustained loss of cooling over many hours, or a severe external event such as an earthquake or the impact of an aircraft, might cause the storage tank to fail and release a significant fraction of its inventory. Such potential events have to be covered in the emergency plans for nuclear fuel reprocessing plants.

16.4 UNCONTROLLED CRITICALITY

16.4.1 General

The process of fission and the conditions under which a chain reaction can occur have been described in Chapter 10. Uncontrolled critical excursions are possible in reactors and in any plant or laboratory in which sufficiently large quantities of fissile materials are handled. The main feature of an uncontrolled criticality is the intense prompt neutron and γ radiation given off during the excursion. If it occurs in an area where there is little or no shielding a very large external hazard results. However, if it occurs in the core of a reactor, the hazard is greatly reduced by the biological shield. In either situation, if the energy released is large enough it can result in an explosive reaction, loss of containment and a release of radioactivity.

There are three approaches to the prevention of criticality when large quantities of fissile material are present:

1. provision of **neutron absorbers**;
2. the use of **safe geometry**; and
3. limitation of quantity (**batching**).

In a reactor, method (1) is the most important while in fuel plants methods (2) and (3) are used either separately or in combination.

16.4.2 Reactors

In a reactor, criticality is maintained by adjusting the position of the control rods (see section 10.3.2). Uncontrolled criticality could potentially occur if the rods failed to enter the core when required or were suddenly ejected from it. The majority of uncontrolled critical excursions that have occurred on reactors have involved low-power experimental facilities, rather than large power reactors. The accidents were, in most cases, caused by a combination of circumstances such as a bad design feature, a mechanical or electrical failure and an operator error.

The most comprehensively investigated and reported accident was on the SL1 reactor at Idaho Falls, USA, in 1961. Following a routine shut-down for maintenance, an operating crew of three men was reassembling the control rod drives in preparation for start-up. The design of the rod drive mechanisms was such that the rods had to be raised manually a few centimetres while they were being connected. It appears that the central control rod was manually withdrawn about 0.5 m causing the reactor to go critical. The energy released caused a violent steam explosion which killed the three operators. Recovery operations were hampered by radiation levels of about 10 Sv/h inside the reactor building owing to fission products released from the core. Very little release of radioactivity from the building occurred even though it had not been designed as a containment. The accident resulted from a serious design fault and inadequate supervision or training of the operators. Modern reactor designs, both experimental and power, attempt to ensure that such events are virtually impossible.

16.4.3 Reactor fuel plants

There are three types of reactor fuel plant, namely, enrichment, fuel fabrication and irradiated fuel reprocessing plants, all of which handle large quantities of fissile material. The material may be in solid form or in solution, the latter form being more hazardous because of the neutron moderation provided by the solvent.

The safe geometry method involves making all process vessels, tanks and pipework of such a shape that their contents cannot go critical. The most efficient shape to produce a critical arrangement is a sphere since in this configuration neutrons are least likely to escape without causing further fission. Conversely, the safest shapes are thin slabs or tall cylinders.

The safe geometry method can also be applied to the handling of fissile materials in solid forms such as billets, rods or plates of fuel. An example of this is the **thin-layer method**. Here, the essential feature is that within a given area all fissile material is stored, processed, transported and generally handled within a certain layer. For example, if the safe thickness for the type of material being handled is 0.15 m, all fissile material would be stored, processed, etc., at a specified height, say between 1.0 m and 1.15 m above floor level. All working surfaces would be 1.0 m high, and trolleys, machines and storage racks would be arranged so that the material always remained in the thin layer.

Batching means that the fissile material is processed through the plant in quantities that are too small to go critical even under the worst geometry. To provide a good margin of safety, batches are usually small enough to ensure safety even if double-batching should occur because of a mechanical or administrative failure. Another important point is that vessels and batches must be adequately spaced to prevent interaction between them.

Whichever method of criticality control is used allowance must be made for contingencies. In particular, the possibility of flooding must be considered because of the moderation and reflection provided by water. Plans for fire-fighting are often complicated by the need to preclude water from the area.

Fuel plant accidents are typified by that which occurred at Los Alamos, New Mexico, USA, in 1958. While an inventory was being taken of plutonium residues, the contents of two tanks were drained into a third tank. The two tanks had each contained a safe quantity but when added they constituted an unsafe quantity. The residues were fairly heavy and settled in the bottom of the tank in a subcritical configuration. However, when the tank was electrically stirred the residues mixed with the solvent which provided neutron moderation and the system went critical. The operator received a fatal dose estimated at 120 Gy.

16.5 PREPLANNING FOR EMERGENCIES

One important result of the TMI accident, mentioned in Section 16.3.3, was that all countries reviewed their preplanned arrangements for nuclear emergencies. In the USA this resulted, among other things, in an increase in the distance from the plant for which detailed preplanning was required. In the UK the review group concluded that the distances did not need to be increased but called for a number of actions to improve the coordination of emergency services and to streamline the decision-making process in the event of an emergency. The Chernobyl accident caused a further re-evaluation of emergency arrangements.

In the two decades since the Chernobyl accident, international organizations such as the EU and national governments and regulatory authorities have adopted an increasingly formal approach to emergency planning and providing information to the public. Increasingly, operators of premises where work with radiation is carried out have been required to carry out formal hazard and risk assessments in order to:

- identify what reasonably practicable measures might be taken to prevent foreseeable accidents and mitigate the consequences of any that might occur;
- provide a structured basis on which to plan for emergencies and provide information to the public;
- supply information to the local authority to enable an off-site plan to be prepared.

In the UK, the Radiation (Emergency Preparedness and Public Information) Regulations (REPPIR) were adopted in 2001 to implement the articles of the 1996 Basic Safety Standards Directive which dealt with intervention in cases of radiological emergencies. REPPIR also implements relevant parts of the 1989 Public Information Directive on informing the general public about health protection measures to be applied and steps to be taken in the event of an emergency.

Preplanning to deal with emergency situations begins at the design stage of any plant, process or experiment. A detailed safety analysis at this stage not only indicates the major hazards but may also enable methods of reducing them to be incorporated in the design. No matter how good the design is, or how many safeguards are provided, there always remains the possibility of an accident and to deal with this eventuality an **emergency organization** is required.

The size of the organization depends very much on the type of plant and the possible scale of the emergency. In a large plant such as a power reactor the organization is quite large and includes representatives from different departments. For example:

Administration department can assist with such matters as transport, liaison with external authorities and other services, and communicating with the media.

Engineering department is responsible for providing rescue and damage control teams, decontamination services and maintaining emergency equipment.

Medical department deals with casualties, radiation or otherwise, and liaises with hospitals and medical authorities.

Health physics department provides monitoring equipment and services and advises on all aspects of radiation protection.

The actions required and the responsibilities of the various parties in the organization are detailed in the **emergency procedures**. This document includes instructions on evacuation, monitoring, communications, re-entry and use of emergency equipment.

The emergency equipment includes rescue equipment, medical equipment, protective clothing, breathing apparatus and monitoring instruments. In the last case, it must be borne in mind that very high radiation and contamination levels may occur and so special high-range instruments are required. In the SL1 accident mentioned earlier the radiation levels encountered by the rescue team were greater than the maximum range of their instruments (5 Gy/h). Instruments extending up to about 50 Gy/h are now available for emergency use.

Finally, the importance of exercising the emergency organization must be emphasized. No matter what the scale of a potential situation, regular exercises remind staff of their actions and responsibilities, test the emergency equipment and highlight shortcomings in the procedures.

SUMMARY OF CHAPTER

Radiological emergency: abnormal or unexpected hazard.

Various levels of severity: local incident, site emergency or public emergency.

Potential causes of radiological emergencies: loss of shielding, loss of containment or criticality – usually as a result of conventional failure.

Detection of situation: vital that an incident is recognized immediately – importance of installed instruments.

Preplanning: begins at design stage and requires detailed safety analysis.

Emergency organization: emergency procedures and equipment. Emergency exercises.

REVISION QUESTIONS

1. What is a radiological emergency and how could such a situation arise?
2. Discuss the importance of rapid detection of the situation and explain how this might be achieved in practice.
3. With particular reference to reactor fuel plants, describe the methods by which the criticality risk is controlled.
4. Write a short set of emergency instructions to apply in the event of a spillage in a small laboratory handling about 100 MBq of a low-toxicity nuclide.

The organization and administration of health physics services

17.1 THE OVERALL PROCESS

The previous chapters of the book have been devoted to explaining the technical concepts and practice of radiation protection. In this final chapter the more general aspects of organization and administrative control are considered.

The process of radiation protection depends on:

1. The establishment of standards for radiation protection.
2. The formulation of regulations and codes of practice to meet the standards.
3. The design and operation of plants or facilities in accordance with the codes.
4. The supervision and continuous review of the whole process.

17.2 STANDARDS, REGULATIONS AND CODES

It has been mentioned in earlier chapters that the radiation protection standards used in most countries are based on the recommendations of the International Commission on Radiological Protection (ICRP). These recommendations are continually reviewed in the light of new evidence from research institutions in many parts of the world. As explained in Chapter 14, countries that are members of the European Union (EU) are subject to the Euratom Treaty and must comply with the standards laid down in the EU Directives on radiation protection. The Directives reflect the thinking and numerical values of the most recent ICRP recommendations.

In the UK, for example, the 1996 Basic Safety Standards Directive was implemented by a comprehensive regulatory framework established under the Health and Safety at Work (HSW) Act. A multi-tiered approach was adopted which comprised:

1. **Regulations,** particularly the *Ionizing Radiations Regulations (1999)*, which specify duties and requirements, dose limits, record-keeping requirements, and so on.
2. An approved code of practice, which explains the detailed application of the regulations in specific areas of work activity and gives guidance on matters of general concern to those involved with ionizing radiations. This code of practice is issued by the Health and Safety Executive (HSE).

3. Guidance notes, published under the auspices of the HSE, which give more detailed advice and guidance on certain topics, taking into account local circumstances. At the plant level, there are usually detailed procedure documents which interpret the requirements of the official regulations in the context of the particular operations being undertaken.

17.3 DESIGN AND OPERATION

Radiation protection in any plant begins at the planning and design stage. This means that the designer must be familiar with the general concepts of radiation hazards and the means of controlling them. In addition, there must be extensive consultation between the designer and various specialists. These could include chemists, physicists, health physicists, fire prevention officers and industrial safety experts.

The need for advance planning applies not only to the design of the plant but also to the methods of operation and maintenance. As a general principle, where an error in operation could result in a serious radiation hazard, engineered safeguards should be provided either to prevent the error or to limit its consequences. For example, for a reactor, the consequences of an operator error are limited by the reactor protection system which would shut down the reactor if the power or temperature exceeded some predetermined value.

The problems of maintenance must also be given careful consideration at the design stage. The sort of situation that should be avoided is the location of equipment which needs frequent maintenance in areas of high radiation. Similarly, the possibility of releases of radioactive contamination as a result of maintenance operations and the implications for plant layout should be considered. All of these aspects are considered as part of a design review process, often called an ALARA (as low as reasonably achievable) review. This involves detailed assessments of the radiological conditions that will arise in the operation of the plant, and of the requirements for access to the various areas and items of equipment for the purposes of operation and maintenance. The major contributions to worker dose and ways of reducing this dose can then be identified. The review usually follows a formal approach addressing a series of issues such as: Can the source terms be reduced by reducing the amount of radioactivity in a part of the system? Can shielding be provided on part or all of the active plant? Can the layout be improved to increase the distance? Can the operating procedures be changed to reduce the amount of access needed? Can maintenance requirements be reduced by careful selection of equipment? Account also needs to be taken of the possibility of abnormal operating conditions and of incidents. The results of such reviews are fed back into the design in an iterative process. In large and complex plants such as reactors or chemical plants, operation and maintenance is usually in accordance with detailed written procedures. These are subject to periodic review.

17.4 SUPERVISION AND REVIEW

Supervision and review of the processes of radiation protection occurs at several levels. At the top level, the ICRP keeps under continuous review the overall philosophy for radiation protection in the light of advancing knowledge and changing circumstances. It also keeps under review information on the biological effects of radiation in order to ensure that its recommendations remain valid.

At the national level, government bodies or regulators maintain a watching brief on the industries for which they have responsibilities. Statistical surveys can be an important component of these reviews. For example, annual reviews of dose statistics broken down into different sectors and occupations can help to reveal trends and identify areas that need special attention. Similarly, event reports and accident statistics can focus attention onto problem areas. At the organizational level, periodic reviews of radiation protection are essential. For example, the preparation of an annual radiological report provides the senior staff responsible for preparing the report with an opportunity to pause and take stock. The report also helps the management to monitor the situation.

At a more detailed level, the radiation protection staff of a facility need to keep under continuous review a whole range of issues. These include:

- the radiological conditions around the facilities, particularly during non-routine operations and maintenance periods;
- the adequacy of the classification of controlled and supervised areas;
- the dose performance of different groups of workers;
- the selection, calibration and maintenance of monitoring equipment; and
- the training of health physics and other staff.

All of these review processes are an important part of the overall process of radiation protection. They ensure that the appropriate safety standards are applied, that regulatory policies and procedures develop with changing circumstances, and that good practice is applied to all aspects of the design and operation of facilities.

17.5 THE HEALTH PHYSICS ORGANIZATION

A Health Physics Department is strictly a service organization. Its function is to advise on all matters relating to radiation safety and to provide personnel and equipment to ensure that safety standards are being met. Its attitude should be constructive in that its staff should try to anticipate problems and suggest alternative approaches rather than waiting for problems to arise and then 'stopping the job'. This presupposes good communications at all levels with other departments.

In general, members of a health physics organization should be independent and not have other duties in which a conflict of interests could occur. This is not always possible in small organizations where health physics duties may be a part-time responsibility, but the job specifications should be carefully constructed to avoid potential conflicts.

The 1996 Basic Safety Standards Directive defines the term 'qualified expert' and establishes requirements for the training, experience and recognition of such experts. An Annex to the Directive gives the topics to be addressed in a basic syllabus for the education in radiation protection of the qualified expert. In addition, it recommends specific topics to be included in the syllabus for five specific areas, i.e. nuclear installations, general industry, research and training, medical applications and accelerators. Surveys within the EU indicate a wide diversity in the approaches of Member States to the training and qualifications of the radiation protection expert. This makes mutual recognition of the qualified expert, as defined in Article 1 of the Basic Safety Standards Directive, difficult between Member States. Steps are being taken to improve this situation, including the creation of a discussion platform to allow for a better harmonization of education and training requirements in the different areas of radiation protection.

In the UK, the **Radiation Protection Advisor (RPA)** is the equivalent term used for the qualified expert as described in the Basic Safety Standards Directive. Under the HSW Act an

RPA has to be appointed by employers whose operations require the designation of **controlled** or **supervised areas** (see Chapter 14). The RPA must have suitable qualifications and experience, which must be notified to the HSE. In addition to the RPA a **radiation protection supervisor (RPS)** should be appointed to provide local supervision. The RPS should be suitably qualified and should have a sound working knowledge of radiological protection in relation to the particular activities for which he or she is appointed. More than one RPA and RPS may be appointed if the range of the duties or the processes involved warrant it.

In addition to the RPA and the RPS, the health physics organization of a large establishment will usually contain technical support staff, health physics foremen, health physics monitors and clerical staff.

The basis of an efficient health physics organization is a sound programme of routine work. This includes:

1. The administration of a personnel monitoring service and the keeping of up-to-date dose records.
2. The performance and recording of routine radiation and contamination surveys in and around controlled areas, and the analysis of the results to observe trends.
3. In collaboration with the Instrument Department, the provision, maintenance and calibration of monitoring equipment.
4. The mustering, testing and recording of all radioactive sources.
5. Provision and regular testing of emergency equipment.

There may be a number of other duties depending on the range of activities and organization of the establishment as a whole; for example:

6. Provision of protective clothing and equipment.
7. Control of radioactive waste and the keeping of records.
8. Making arrangements for the medical examinations of classified workers.

Then there are, of course, the day-to-day operational aspects that provide much of the interest. These involve the provision of advice and monitoring during special or non-routine operations in which significant radiological hazards could arise.

17.6 DOCUMENTS AND REPORTS

Various records and reports are required to be kept either because of statutory obligation or in accordance with a code of practice.

The **Health Record** is a record of all medical examinations performed on an employee while they are a category A worker. The records for a particular person are required to be preserved for 50 years after the last entry.

The **Source Record** contains information on all radioactive sources and the dates and results of all leakage tests. Retention period is 2 years after the last entry.

The **Instrument Record** is used to record details and results of tests of all instruments used for health physics purposes. Retention period is 2 years after the last entry.

Radiation dose records are required to be kept in respect of all classified workers and to be retained until the person reaches 75 years of age or for 50 years after the last entry, whichever is the greatest. Under the HSE regulatory framework an approved dosimetry service has to be used for the assessment of personal dose and the retention of dose records.

Each record includes the worker's national insurance number, and the worker has the right to examine his or her dose record. When a worker changes jobs, he or she will be given a termination record detailing the current dose status (purely for information), and the new employer will seek such a record from his or her own approved laboratory, which will carry out the necessary consultation. The 1999 *Ionizing Radiations Regulations* introduced a new requirement on employers to ensure that any outside workers employed by them are provided with individual **radiation passbooks** and that these passbooks are kept up to date. When the worker moves to a different employer, he or she transfers the passbook to that employer. This system helps to ensure that the doses received by itinerant workers are kept within the statutory dose limits.

Survey Records, containing the results of routine radiation and contamination surveys, are usually retained for at least 2 years.

Reports of unusual occurrences: all unusual occurrences that result in or could have resulted in an abnormal radiation dose should be fully investigated. The reports are normally preserved for at least 50 years.

Waste disposal records are preserved indefinitely, in particular those records showing the location of buried solid waste.

17.7 TRAINING

The safety records of industries that use sources of ionizing radiation, particularly the atomic energy industry, are generally very good. This is, to a large extent, the result of their positive attitude to staff training. The legislation and codes of practice require that all persons exposed to radiation in the course of their work should be given training in the hazards and the means of controlling them. This may vary from a short talk on the function of personal dosimeters and an outline of local rules to a detailed course in health physics, depending on the nature of the plant and the duties of those involved.

Specialist courses are necessary for health physics personnel. Large establishments often run their own training courses for health physics monitors and technicians, while others make use of courses run by colleges or universities or by specialist organizations. In the UK, the Radiological Protection Division of the Health Protection Agency organizes a number of courses on radiological protection, ranging from short familiarization courses to advanced courses for specialist health physicists. In North America and in Europe there are well-established summer schools that aim to provide intensive refresher courses for professionals in radiological protection.

A most important aspect of training for all health physics personnel is plant familiarization, that is, instruction in the processes and engineering aspects of the plant on which they will be working. An understanding of the plant is essential if proper advice is to be given and a constructive attitude maintained.

SUMMARY OF CHAPTER

ALARA review: a formal review of the design and/or operation of a plant.
Considerations in routine radiation protection: standards, regulations and codes, design and operation of plant, health physics organization, documentation and reporting.
Health Record: record of all medical examinations while person is a classified worker.
Source Record: contains information on all radioactive sources with dates and results of all leakage tests.

Instrument Record: record of tests on all health physics instruments, retained 2 years after last entry.

Radiation dose records: for classified workers, retention period 50 years after last entry.

Survey Records: usually retained for at least 2 years.

Reports of unusual occurrences: retained for at least 50 years.

Waste disposal records: preserved indefinitely.

Training: radiation protection, plant familiarization.

Appendix A: Relationship of units

Radiological quantity	Old unit	SI Unit	Relationship between units		
Activity of a radioactive material	The curie 1 Ci = 3.7 × 10^{10} dis/s	The becquerel 1 Bq = 1 dis/s 10^3 Bq = 1 kilobecquerel (kBq) 10^6 Bq = 1 megabecquerel (MBq) 10^9 Bq = 1 gigabecquerel (GBq) 10^{12} Bq = 1 terabecquerel (TBq) 10^{15} Bq = 1 petabecquerel (PBq) 10^{18} Bq = 1 exabecquerel (EBq)	1 Bq = 2.7 × 10^{-11} Ci 1 kBq = 2.7 × 10^{-8} Ci 1 MBq = 2.7 × 10^{-5} Ci = 27 μCi 1 GBq = 27 mCi 1 TBq = 27 Ci 1 PBq = 27 kCi 1 EBq = 27 MCi	1 μCi = 37 kBq 1 mCi = 37 MBq 1 Ci = 37 GBq 10^3 Ci = 37 TBq 10^6 Ci = 37 PBq 10^9 Ci = 37 EBq	
Absorbed dose	The rad 1 rad = 0.01 J/kg	The gray 1 Gy = 1 J/kg 1 Gy = 10^3 mGy = 10^6 μGy	1 μGy = 0.1 mrad 1 mGy = 100 mrad 1 Gy = 100 rad	1 mrad = 10 μGy 1 rad = 10 mGy 100 rad = 1 Gy	
Equivalent dose	The rem 1 rem = 1 rad × Q Q is the quality factor	The sievert 1 Sv = 1 Gy × w_R 1 Sv = 10^3 mSv = 10^6 μSv w_R is the radiation weighting factor	1 μSv = 0.1 mrem 1 mSv = 100 mrem 1 Sv = 100 rem	1 mrem = 10 μSv 1 rem = 10 mSv 100 rem = 1 Sv	

Appendix B: Answers to numerical questions

Chapter 1

2. 27, 27, 33.
3. 1; 1/1840; 1; $+1, -1, 0$.

Chapter 2

2. (a) $^{234}_{90}$Th; (b) $^{3}_{2}$He; (c) $^{62}_{28}$Ni.
4. 2.3 min.
5. (a) 5 MBq; (b) 0.75 MBq; (c) 1300 MBq; (d) 1 MBq.

Chapter 3

5. 2.65×10^{7} n/(m²s).
6. $-84\,\mu$Sv.
7. 1.2 mSv.

Chapter 5

2. 2.20 mSv/year $\times$ 30 years $=$ 66 mSv.

Chapter 6

3. 150 mSv, 500 mSv.
5. 40 mSv.
6. 400 mSv, 167 mSv, 167 mSv, 400 mSv.

Chapter 8

2. 10 h, 2.5 μSv/h.
3. 225 μSv/h, 3 m.
4. 6 m.
5. 200 μSv/h.

Chapter 9

1. 11.1 mSv.
2. 312.5 Bq.
4. $4 \times 10^4 \, \text{Bq/m}^2$.
5. $1.67 \times 10^4 \, \text{Bq/m}^3$.

Chapter 15

2. 1970 Bq.
4. Maximum β-energy 1.71 MeV, half-life 14.3 days, phosphorus-32.
6. $382 \pm 3.4 \, \text{counts/min}$.
7. 1.9, 1.2, 0.85 and 0.6 m.

Bibliography

GENERAL REFERENCES

The publications of the International Commission on Radiological Protection (ICRP) are a key source of information on many aspects of radiation protection. They include both recommendations and topical reports prepared by task groups. See http://www.icrp.org

Turner, J. E. (1995) *Atoms, Radiation and Radiation Protection*, 2nd edn. Chichester: Wiley and Sons.

This is a comprehensive book aimed at postgraduates and professional health physicists.

CHAPTERS 1 AND 2

Blin-Stoyle, R. J. (1991) *Nuclear and Particle Physics*. London: Chapman & Hall.

This book aims to provide a clear, concise introduction to both nuclear and particle physics, including extensive problem sets and answers.

Jelly, N. A. (1990) *Fundamentals of Nuclear Physics*. Cambridge: Cambridge University Press.

This textbook is designed to provide a thorough understanding of the principal features of nuclei, nuclear decays and nuclear reactions.

CHAPTER 3

Attix, F. H. (1986) *Introduction to Radiological Physics and Radiation Dosimetry*. Chichester: Wiley and Sons.

A straightforward presentation of the broad concepts underlying radiological physics and radiation dosimetry for the graduate level student.

CHAPTER 4

International Commission on Radiation Units and Measurements (1993) *ICRU Report No. 51. Quantities and Units in Radiation Protection Dosimetry*. Washington DC: ICRU.

The ICRU has published numerous reports on detailed aspects of radiation dosimetry and radiation quantities. See www.icru.org

Schull, W. J. (1995) *Effects of Atomic Radiation: A Half-Century of Studies from Hiroshima to Nagasaki*. New York: Alan R. Liss, Inc.

This study of the biological consequences of exposure to atomic radiation incorporates 50 years of data based on long-term studies of atomic bomb survivors.

United Nations Scientific Committee on the Effects of Atomic Radiation (UNSCEAR) (2000) *Sources and Effects of Ionising Radiation*. New York: United Nations.

UNSCEAR (2001) *Hereditary Effects of Radiation*. New York: United Nations.
See http://www.unscear.org

CHAPTER 5

Eisenbud, M. (1987) *Environmental Radioactivity: From Natural, Industrial and Military Sources*, 3rd edn. New York: Academic Press, Inc.
A systematic account is given of the behaviour of radioactive substances in the environment. Topics covered include physical and biological transport mechanisms, sources of environmental radio-activity and experience.
Watson, S. J. *et al.* (2005) *Ionising Radiation Exposure of the UK Population: 2005 Review, Health Protection Agency Report HPA-RPD-001*. London: Health Protection Agency.
See also the UNSCEAR report mentioned for Chapter 4.

CHAPTER 6

International Commission on Radiological Protection (1991) *Publication 60: Recommendations of the ICRP*. London: Elsevier.
See http://www.icrp.org

CHAPTER 7

Attix, F. H. (1986) *Introduction to Radiological Physics and Radiation Dosimetry*. Chichester: Wiley and Sons.
Hallenbeck, W. H. (1994) *Radiation Protection*. Ann Arbor: Lewis.

CHAPTERS 8 AND 9

International Commission on Radiological Protection (1998) *Publication 75. General Principles for Radiation Protection of Workers*. London: Elsevier
See also the ICRP Publications listed under Chapter 6.
International Commission on Radiological Protection (1994) *Publication 67: Age-dependent Doses To Members of The Public from Intake of Radionuclides: Part 2, Ingestion Dose Coefficients*. London: Elsevier.
International Commission on Radiological Protection (1995) *Publication 68: Dose Coefficients for Intakes of Radionuclides by Workers*. London: Elsevier.
International Commission on Radiological Protection Publication 72, Age-dependent doses to members of the public from intake of radionuclides: Part 5 – compilation of ingestion and inhalation dose coefficients. *Annals of the ICRP*, **26**(1), 1996.
International Commission on Radiological Protection (2003) *Publication 89: Basic Anatomical and Physiological Data for Use in Radiological Protection: Reference Values*. London: Elsevier.
The International Atomic Energy Agency (IAEA) is a major publisher in the fields of radiation protection and nuclear energy. The publications include standards and guides, technical reports and scientific reviews. See http://www.iaea.org
    Among the documents of interest are:

International Atomic Energy Agency (1963) *A Basic Toxicity Classification for Radionuclides. Technical Reports Series No. 15.* Vienna: IAEA.

International Atomic Energy Agency (1976) *Design of and equipment for Hot Laboratories, IAEA Proceedings Series STI/PUB/436.* Vienna: IAEA.

This book describes the requirements for containment, shielding, ventilation, fire protection, criticality control, waste management and safety in operations in radioactive facilities. It includes contributions on the latest developments in these areas, emphasis being placed on the safety features of planning and design.

International Atomic Energy Agency (1996) *International Basic Safety Standards for Protection Against Ionizing Radiation and for the Safety of Radiation Sources.* Vienna: IAEA.

CHAPTER 10

Glasstone, S., Sesonske, A. (1994) *Nuclear Reactor Engineering*, 4th edn. Dordrecht: Kluwer Academic Publishers.

This is a sound textbook which covers the fundamental scientific and engineering principles of nuclear reactor systems. The aspects considered in detail include nuclear reactions, reactor theory, control of reactors, reactor materials and fuels, radiation protection, reactor safeguards and shielding.

Shultis, J. K., Faw, R. E. (2000) *Radiation Shielding.* La Grange Park: American Nuclear Society.

CHAPTER 11

Bayliss, C., Langley, K. (2003) *Nuclear Decommissioning, Waste Management and Environmental Remediation.* Oxford: Butterworth-Heineman.

International Atomic Energy Agency (1994) *Classification of Radioactive Waste: A Safety Guide* Vienna: IAEA.

Saling, J. H., (ed), Tang, Y. S., Fentiman, A. W. (1990) *Radioactive Waste Management.* London: Taylor and Francis.

CHAPTERS 12 AND 13

Martin, C. J., Dendy, P. P., Corbett, R. H. (2003) *Medical Imaging and Radiation Protection for Medical Students and Clinical Staff.* London: British Institute of Radiology.

Adler, A. M., Carlton, R. R. (1993) *Introduction to Radiography and Patient Care.* Philadelphia: W. B. Saunders.

Merrick, M. V. (1997) *Essentials of Nuclear Medicine.* Berlin: Springer-Verlag.

CHAPTER 14

Organization for Economic Co-operation and Development Nuclear Energy Agency (1972) *Nuclear Legislation. An Analytical Study of Regulations Governing Nuclear Installations and Radiation Protection.* Paris: OECD Nuclear Energy Agency.

Organization for Economic Co-operation and Development Nuclear Energy Agency (1980) *Description of Licensing Systems and Inspection of Nuclear Installations.* Paris: OECD Nuclear Energy Agency.

Organization for Economic Co-operation and Development Nuclear Energy Agency (1990) *Nuclear Legislation: Third Party Liability.* Paris: OECD Nuclear Energy Agency.

CHAPTER 15

Brown, B. (1963) *Experimental Nucleonics.* London: Iliffe Books.
The first half of this book is an account of the general principles of radiation detection and measurement. This is followed by detailed notes on a series of experiments suitable for a course in radiation protection.

CHAPTER 16

International Atomic Energy Authority (2002*) Preparedness and response for a nuclear or radiological emergency. Safety Standards Series No. GS-R-2.* Vienna: IAEA.

International Commission on Radiological Protection (1984) *Publication 63. Principles for intervention for protection of the public in a radiological emergency.* London: Elsevier.

Index

Note: page numbers in *italics* refer to tables; page numbers in **bold** refer to figures or examples.